THE SISTERHOOD OF
S.W.E.A.T.

Strong
Women
Empowering
Achieving
Together
#SOS

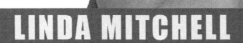

LINDA MITCHELL

To contact the author, visit
www.chickfit.me

ISBN # 978-0-9970306-0-0
Printed in the United States of America

DEDICATION

To my father, who believed in me, was my best friend,
and the most positive man I have ever known.

To my husband, for believing in me and pushing me beyond
what I thought I could be or do. I would never have done this without all
of your hard work which has enabled me to live my dreams.

ACKNOWLEDGEMENTS

To all of my S.W. E. A. T. sisters - Without you, there would be no sisterhood. I enjoy sharing burpees with you before breakfast, before bedtime, and just about any time. But most of all, thank you for your brilliance and friendship.

To Cathy Savage, for reflecting all that is good in this world. You are a true entrepreneur, leader, coach, and beautiful human being whom I truly look up to. I look forward to learning and being inspired by you for many years to come. www.cathysavagefitness.com

To Kate McKay, author of *Living Sexy Fit*, for being a light in the darkness and for helping to set me on a clear path to success. www.kate-mckay.com

To Sharon Polsky, WBFF Pro and owner of Pole Position Fitness. Thank you for being so solid and kicking my butt when I need it. I have learned so much from you. You sincerely ROCK, girl, and I love you for it. www.polepositionfitness.com

To Sarah Lyons, for being an outstanding artist and photographer. Thank you for always bringing the beauty from the inside to shine on the outside. You have a gift for making a woman feel comfortable, beautiful, and free in front of your lens. www.picturegroovephotography.com

To Michael, Jake, and Tiffany, for putting up with your over-the-top zealous, fitness enthusiast and health nut mom. Thanks for your beautiful grown up lives, your greatest gift. I am so proud to be your mother.

To Jake Mitchell - Your talent and drive amaze me and I'm proud to call you my son. Thanks for all of your help editing and your insight. Thanks for trying out all of my healthy experiments.

To Michael Nicholson - Thanks for always being a sounding board. Your support and wise advice has clearly brought me to where I am at this very moment.

To my longtime friend Amy Schrock Green, who has been by my side through thick and thin and the ups and downs. Amy always has my back and truly knows me.

To my husband, Tracy - There would be no book if it weren't for your love and support. I love that you can always make me laugh. Thanks for always being the voice of reason. You are my rock.

To my mother, Margie, who introduced me to healthy and fit living through her beautiful example. I can still hear the words of my father, "I'm such a fortunate young man that your mother is such a good cook."

To Debbie Haumesser - Thank you for always supporting me and being my cheerleader. Thanks a ton for all of your help fine tuning the book.

SISTERHOOD OF S.W.E.A.T. CHICKMONIALS

Healing Through Fitness

This is a book about healing through fitness and being healthy. It's not all about the way you look, it's about the way you feel and the vitality that you are able to bring to life. It's about being able to do the things you want to do because you're fit and healthy on the inside and the outside. The following stories are from individuals whose lives, bodies, and minds have transformed and healed through fitness.

"I never would have dreamed that I would be a person who says, "I can't wait for my workout." One year ago, after delivering my second child within a two year period, I found myself fifty plus pounds over my pre-babies weight. I had a history of being overweight when I was younger and was terrified of returning to that place in my life. Weight struggles have been an issue with me since I was in the sixth grade. As I started to gain weight, my self-esteem began to decrease. By the time that I hit my junior year in high school I weighed about 190 pounds and was on the receiving end of many weight jokes. It affected my high school years in that I did not have many friends and was very self-conscious. In between my junior and senior year, I managed to drop quite a bit of weight and was able to maintain but still found myself very self-conscious about my appearance. Fast forward to the age of thirty-five. I had just given birth to my second child and was weighing in at 205 pounds. I was starting to find myself slipping into that pit of despair and self-loathing that I experienced in high school. That is when I met Linda Mitchell. I signed up for one of her boot camp classes and that is where my fitness journey started. Linda was able to not only help me shed some unwanted pounds but she also was able to show me how to live an active healthy lifestyle. Within a matter of four months she had decreased my body fat significantly with the use of nutritional coaching and workout routines. In four months I shed over forty pounds and dropped four pant sizes. I am sitting, writing this letter, sixty pounds lighter, five pant sizes smaller, and in the best physical shape I have ever been in. I am doing workouts now that I never thought I'd be able to do. Linda and the close-knit group of girls I work out with have made the most tremendous and positive impact on my life and I will be eternally grateful. I can't express how good it feels to hear people tell me how nice I look and comment on the progress I have made. I am in the best shape I have ever been in and I feel great. Fitness has become my way of life and I get very cranky when I miss workouts. Being healthy and fit has empowered me to take on challenges that I never thought that I could achieve. In August of 2014, I participated in my first Mud Guts and Glory obstacle race and in October of the same year I competed in my first Fitness Universe Competition. Now I am looking forward to participating in the Spartan Race with Linda Mitchell and the other fine ladies of the ChickFit team!"

~Kathie Koch

"Joining Linda was never about losing the extra pounds I had gained since high school or dropping the number I regularly read on my bathroom scale. For me, joining Linda was about something much bigger. I wanted a healthy lifestyle that matched how I finally felt about myself.

Unfortunately, my childhood was a dark one. I grew up in a divided home with poisonous step parents on either side. Many forms of abuse were common and very regular, in fact, daily. I developed little to no self-worth and maintained a constant state of "survivor mode." I definitely had a chip on my shoulder and once I turned eighteen, I moved out. I figured I could take care of myself and finally be in control. I was wrong. My childhood didn't teach me how to care for myself or how to be in a healthy relationship. I quickly developed several drug addictions as my defense mechanism to escape reality. I became addicted to cocaine, alcohol, psychedelics, marijuana, and anything I could get. You name it, I did it.

My love life was just as disastrous. Because I didn't grow up in a loving home, I didn't know what love looked like and naturally, I was attracted to what I did know....poison. After my divorce at twenty-two, my many vices increased in intensity. I started hanging out with an even rougher crowd. By age twenty-six, I didn't recognize myself. I had no idea how I had become the disgruntled woman I saw in the mirror. I knew I had to change.

I began therapy and it was quickly revealed how my dark past was affecting my decision making and why I chose drugs and alcohol as comfort. My slews of neglectful, unhealthy, and unfulfilling relationships were a result of me not valuing myself. In general, everything became clear. I became clean and started facing the past I had been running so hard from. It was an incredibly sad and difficult time in my life.
After being completely clean for six months, I decided it was time to focus on a different aspect of my health. Therapy had done wonders and gave me the tools I needed to care for myself, but I wanted more. I had been given a new foundation to build upon and wanted to be the best version of myself I could. It was time to focus on my physical self. I knew I needed support and to be surrounded by healthy minded people. I wanted a sisterhood.

Linda's Sisterhood of S.W.E.A.T. was exactly what I was looking for and needed. I've never felt so great and healthy in all aspects in my life. I absolutely love the atmosphere she has created. It's supportive, fun, and continuously challenging. There's absolutely no judgment from anyone. Everyone has their reasons for joining and we're all there with a similar goal, to be better. Whether it's to be slimmer, stronger, faster, or just healthy, Linda can help. Sisterhood of S.W.E.A.T. has given me another reason to stay clean and healthy as well as to continue to work on myself. I am proud of who I am today and how far I've come. I finally love the path I'm on!
Thank you, Linda!"

~Corinne Pease

"Deciding to join Linda on this fitness journey was one of the scariest things I had ever done. Let me just say that I am not an athlete. I am forty-seven years old and have never played a sport or been very active. I'm the type of person that enjoys being "comfortable," not pushing myself to eat the right thing or do more than just the least amount of exercise. That kind of lifestyle tends to catch up with you at some point, and I didn't like the way I felt or the size I had become. I came across this quote by Pastor Rick Warren. He said, "God created it. Jesus died for it. The Spirit lives in it. I'd better take care of it." This made me stop and think that I better start taking care of my health.

So I went to my first workout beyond nervous and that is when I met Linda. I made it through the workout and I was amazed that even though it challenged me, Linda made it doable. She was patient, kind, and loving. I wasn't sore until the next day but that was overshadowed by how accomplished and pumped up I felt. Linda always knows when to push you and when to hold back. I could not have done this without Linda's encouragement and clear instructions. I have done eating plans before and some exercise but Linda puts everything together in this unbelievable package that works! She always works out with me and gives me tips on food choices. On top of that, her enthusiasm is contagious!

I had read countless Pinterest blogs that would say "Do these 10 things and you'll lose 10 lbs.," or, "Eat these 5 things and you'll be fit." What I found was that I had to jump in with both feet, trust God to give me the strength and courage, have someone that could teach me and hold me accountable through the process, and to be committed whole heartedly. The best part about this journey is that I didn't have to wait long before I saw results. Not just results on the outside (although that was amazing!), but results on the inside. I'm loving that I am taking care of this body/temple that God gifted me with forty-seven years ago. I'm proud of the courageous, strong, brave woman that I have been all along the way, but now I can feel and see it!"

~Michelle Kappa

"I stumbled across Linda Mitchell and the sisterhood of ChickFit seven weeks postpartum. After having my first baby and being fortunate enough to have six months of maternity leave, I found myself extremely motivated to get my body back before returning to work. I had hit a plateau and knew that without someone pushing and supporting me to meet my own personal goals, it would be a struggle. Not only did I lose 65 pounds before returning to work, I also made lifestyle changes in my fitness and diet. Linda is a great motivator and challenges us all to always strive to push our personal boundaries to new heights. Although the workouts are tough, Linda and the women at ChickFit always make them fun for us all! Because of Linda, not only am I loving my new role as a mommy, but I am also loving myself–it does not get much better than that!"

~Megan Adams

"What had I gotten myself into?! In mid-August, at Voice of America Metropark, I bought a fifteen class Groupon for a boot camp. I was 270 pounds, in a size 22-24, and apprehensive. I had just had surgery on my right knee and the surgeon said I needed to lose weight and strengthen my knees. I was working on the weight loss with my doctor, but I had plateaued over the summer. I knew I needed to do something different, but what had I gotten myself into?! Linda Mitchell, our boot camp instructor, kept saying to me, "Only do what you can. Just keep moving. Try for a little more every time." After the first time, I was not sure there was going to be a next time. *But what the heck, I bought the classes, right?* TRX was easy to modify and the exercises and the Kangoo Boots were fun. I hadn't run in years. In the boots, I could jog a little even though the walkers were passing me. Then Linda announced the Perfect Ten Challenge—ten weeks of following Linda's nutrition plan and 3-4 workouts per week. Could I ever get into my jeans again? I had to take a chance. Well, it worked! The weight and inches just started falling off! As of February, I am now down ninety-four pounds. I am wearing size 14-16 and I have my life back. I can do things around the house and keep up with my kids, instead of collapsing on the couch after work. But, wait! This is the best part! I love roller coasters, but for years I was unable to ride them because the seatbelts wouldn't latch. It was humiliating to have spent time in line just to have to walk away in front of all the other riders. This year, I have a season pass to Kings Island in my purse, just waiting for April 27th, the opening day. I'm going to ride every rollercoaster in the park, over and over again. I'm going to wear out my kids! There is not a ride I can't fit in! Thank you, Linda! You have helped me become a better mother, wife, and person."

~Lisa Babcock

"As I sat down to write this testimony I thought of all the reasons I joined ChickFit. I was praying day and night for God to lead me to a gym that empowered women and helped them to be all God had created them to be. Like God always does, he led me right to Linda Lu and her amazing studio filled with some awesome ladies!

Linda's gym is not like most gyms where everyone is staring at you, wondering what this out of shape woman is doing at the gym (*hellllllo, I am here to get in shape*). It is literally a place of sisterhood. We cheer each other on, laugh about the troubles of our days, and even share with complete strangers how we got to this point in our lives. It is freeing on many levels day-in and day-out.

I was afraid at first, thinking I would look stupid, thinking I was so out of shape, thinking that I definitely didn't have what it takes to get through the workouts. I was very wrong. With God's strength, Linda's motivation, the other women in the class cheering me on, and much prayer, I kept coming back. With every step I took I could feel myself growing stronger and stronger.

Today, I am much stronger and feel I can do any workout that Linda puts in front of me. I eat clean 90% of the time now and Linda is continuously giving me tips on how I can make eating clean enjoyable! Even though my fitness journey has just begun, I have improved so much and can't wait to see where it takes me. I am so thankful that God led me to this gym, these wonderful women, and Linda Lu! I have gained so much strength and confidence training with her."

~Shyla Gardner

FOREWORD
by Kate McKay

In my over thirty years in the fitness and wellness industry, I have met hundreds of women who have faced many challenges to get fit and attain the life they desire. Linda Mitchell is truly one who stands out boldly above the pack.

My colleague and friend Linda Mitchell personifies the power of redemption, facing domestic abuse, financial hardship and loss and to come out on the other side a courageous role model for other women. Linda is a beacon to others of the possibility to succeed and live a life of their dreams.

When I first met Linda in 2011 at a fitness competition, she was already blazing the trail in the fitness industry through her many wins as a competitive athlete, author and personal trainer. Linda was a powerful presence; however, through my fine-tuned skills as a coach, I instinctually knew as soon as I met her, that her success had not come easy. There was vulnerability behind the tough fitness girl and the six pack abs that drew me in. It was only after our first phone consultation about growing her business and getting this book written, that the true details of her challenges came to light. Her story inspired me and I am sure it will inspire you too.

The book you are holding is not only a fantastic tool to get fit and feel more healthy and alive. It is also a book that will empower you to claim your strength and power as well as shed light on how you too can share your own story, for it is through own personal stories that our allegiance as Sisters of Sweat will be sealed.

As you read this phenomenal book, you too can begin the process of fully honoring your own story, for it is by sharing our struggles that we can truly heal and begin to put our health and hotness center stage!

Linda is deeply committed to empowering other women, to celebrating their strength through physical fitness and, most of all, to helping women realize that our past does not need to define us. We are capable of so much more.

With the help of this book, I am convinced you too can embrace your most courageous self and become your most fit and fabulous, no matter your age, race or socio-economics. You deserve all that you desire. It is now your time to go out and get it. We believe in you!

Kate McKay
The Master Motivator
Author of "Living Sexy Fit…at any age"
www.kate-mckay.com
Newburyport, MA.

TABLE OF CONTENTS

Introduction

It's not what you go through in life but what you decide to do about it. I'm a prime example of how bad things can happen to good people. Looking back, I'm thankful for what I've gone through and where I've ended up. I was once in a physically abusive relationship in which I feared for my life. I was raised in church and divorce was not encouraged. I did everything I could to make the marriage work until one day I realized that this was not what God expected of me. This was not the life God had created for me to live. I made the choice to leave and salvage the three good things that were worth saving: my son, my daughter, and myself.

Leaving was scary. I feared for my life and I had to figure out how I was going to survive on my own with two children. Although I graduated high school in the top ten % of my class, at the time, I had never worked full time and only had a high school education. Though the odds were stacked against me, I knew that I would do what it took to make it for my children. I often thought that digging ditches for a living would be better than living the life I had.

After I left my situation, I attended a meeting for abused women. I quickly realized that I had two choices: I could either live my life dwelling on the past or I could go on and make a better future for my children and myself. I knew one thing for sure: I didn't want to live out my tragedy for the rest of my life.

I decided not to dwell on what happened to me or to spend time feeling sorry for myself. I worked very hard and learned to make better choices.

Although the situation seemed hopeless at first, before I knew it, I progressed and began to really thrive. You see, I did a few important things to make a life change: I took ownership of what had happened, decided not to dwell on the past, and I did something about it. I became stronger from my experience. I no longer lived in fear or felt intimidation. I now had something very important. For the first time, I had personal freedom and the confidence that comes from staring fear in the face and saying, "No, I'm done being the victim." I became a victor by not complaining about my situation, blaming him, or justifying bad behavior.

My heart and mission is for women. Although my situation was extreme, I see so many women out there living their life in a box, being controlled by others, and not living the life they were meant to live. I'm here to tell you that you can have the life of your dreams; you just have to be courageous and brave enough to go after it. Somewhere along the line, you have to say, "I'm worthy of having the life I want. I believe in myself."

I never planned on becoming the poster child for abused women. Talking about the past is painful and something I'd rather forget. My hope in bringing this to the forefront is that my story helps someone else out there and raises awareness. I want to shine a light on what is hiding in the dark. Just last night I went to dinner for the first time with some of my husband's friends from Europe and as we began talking and getting to know one another, our stories unfolded to be very similar. Here, Vivian lives in a far away part of the world, in another country and culture, yet her story mirrored the abuse I suffered. Now, for both of us, it is twenty-three years later and we are living happy, productive lives. We were the lucky ones, yet there are so many people out there in these types of situations and it just breaks my heart. This morning, another post (by a lady named Emma) went viral. Emma had a black eye and told her story with many tears to those that would listen and lend an ear. She was from Ireland yet her story mirrored mine. So I am reminded yet again that this is still going on in all parts of the world and that it is a universal problem.

Maybe you can say this is more than an abuse problem. It's a belief problem. What you believe about yourself is pretty powerful. It's also a boundary problem. Be independent enough that you can walk away from somebody that continually violates serious physical and emotional boundaries in your relationship. If you are out there and you are afraid that you can't make it on your own, I'm here to tell you to be strong. Talk to your friends and loved ones and find support. Walk away and never look back. You can do this. As soon as you kick the abuse to the curb, your life will be better. You may be with a partner that isn't striking you physically, but emotional abuse can be far worse. You can't see the marks but the abuse feels the same. You deserve to live a better life, one that is free from fear. You may be surprised to find out that this is a book about health and fitness. When you are going through any type of relationship drama struggle, abuse, or other stress, it wreaks havoc on your health. It doesn't matter what you're eating or how much you're exercising, stress can be a silent killer. Working out and eating right helps relieve stress but sometimes you have to work on having healthy relationships too. True fitness is all encompassing and reaches into every area of your life.

My mantra for personal freedom: I give myself permission to live free, unencumbered or shackled by the insecurities of another. The pursuit of happiness is my God given right. Jealousy and envy are poison and anyone who drinks them is unwelcome in my life. I free myself now to live an unburdened life, full of laughter, smiles, and happiness. I'm stepping out in faith to live the life I know that God meant for me to live, fearless and unafraid.

I can remember when I lived in North Dakota and I really hadn't decided what I wanted to do with my life yet. I was raising two small children and at the age of twenty, I was a baby myself. My husband at the time was in the Air Force. There wasn't much to do on the Air Force base; we were basically snowed in most of the winter and it was very cold, fifty degrees below most days. You definitely did not want to forget your gloves or you would have frostbitten hands for the entire winter. The cold was so extreme that the Airbase had installed units everywhere that we literally had to plug our cars into in order for them to start. There really wasn't much around except for rolling hills and a town about thirty minutes away. It was there, in the little town of Minot, that I really learned how to survive, make my own fun, and become creative. Twelve months after moving to Minot, I gave birth. I named my first born son Michael Ryan after the Archangel and it means "who is like God."

Soon after Michael was born, I went to an exercise class based on Jane Fonda methodology. Aerobics, leotards, and leg warmers were all the rage. I remember that after the first class I thought my stomach muscles had died and went to Heaven. I could barely make it through just one workout. I like to be challenged so I decided to go back for more. In the next class, which was only my second class, I did the best I could to keep up and the instructor told me how impressed she was and that she would be leaving in six months. Would I like to take over her class? Unlike now, where you need to be trained and highly knowledgeable, back in the day you were just elected. By the time she left, I was trained and ready to go. By then, I'd found out I was pregnant with my next child. Yep, that's right, I began as a pregnant instructor. Always one for a challenge, I taught until I knew I could teach no more and that was the day I went into labor. I had a beautiful baby girl. We named her Tiffany Dawn. Tiffany means "in the appearance of God" and Dawn means, well, she was born at the crack of dawn. Dawn suited her. She was always an early bird. My father said that I now had a millionaire's family, a healthy boy and girl.

When I first got started I taught classes on the Airbase. I remember thinking then how great it would be to exercise and be able to teach. I had heard of someone who had a studio in Hollywood, California for the stars. (This was before people really thought about fitness as being much of a career choice.) I thought that it would be awesome to be able to do this all day long for a living. It would be a dream come true to have my own fitness studio and be able to do what I love. Like I said, there wasn't much to do in North Dakota and I had two small children to care for and support so it wasn't like I could go traipsing around the countryside willy-nilly. One snowed-in morning, I was at home watching Good Morning America and on came fitness expert, Joanie

Greggains. She was just so funny and her workouts were so hard that she soon became a fast favorite. I began to work out at home with her every week. I remember thinking, "I don't have much going on now, but maybe if I practice I'll get better at this and be able to do it for a living."

My first teaching gig as the pregnant instructor was at the military recreation center. I taught a floor work Pilates type workout with some cardio interspersed and my classes were packed to the gills. A new gal came along while I was in my heyday and she was teaching Fitness Fantasia which was a Jazzercise type workout. I thought it looked interesting so I had her come to my class and show me some of her choreography. I had never done that type of workout and I'm pretty sure I looked like I had two left feet. She proceeded to tell me after working with me for approximately fifteen minutes that I would never have a career in fitness. I guess thirty career years later, I proved her wrong. This wasn't the first time I had tried my hand at dance. When I was thirteen, I worked with a Cincinnati ballet dancer one afternoon and she informed me that I'd never make it as a ballerina. One thing about me is if you tell me I can't, I will. My class is more athletic style which suits the mainstream population because let's face it, most of us didn't grow up to be ballerinas.

Since that time, I have taken every workshop, training, certification, summit, internship, and convention regardless of where it was located with the very best of the best. I have taught, coached, and competed in everything under the sun such as step aerobics, personal training, kickboxing, water aerobics, Reebok slide, boxing on bags, spinning, Zumba, Shaun-T's dance boot camp S.T.R.I.D.E., Hip-Hop Hustle, Pi-Yo, Turbo-Kick, low-impact and high-impact aerobics, TRX training, kangaroo jumps, rebounding, coached running, yoga, and my overall favorite, boot camp. I went on to train instructors and coordinate in gyms for over twenty-five years before creating my own brand.

One of my strengths is that I'm an activator. I don't let the dust settle under my feet. I have flown to California more times than I can count to "Train the Trainer" with Beth Shaw, the owner and creator of YogaFit. I am certified in YogaFit levels 1-5 as well as Yoga Butt and Yoga Anatomy. I had the great opportunity to work with international fitness celebrity Janis Saffel, ESPN fitness pro Pepper Von, and take classes from Tae Bo creator Billy Blanks. I have been known to discover a new fitness craze, hop on a plane, and two days later be flying to New York learning how to do plyo-glide with Mario Godiva, and then implementing what I learned from him the minute I jump off the plane. When I wanted to take running coaching I flew to Ontario, Canada to learn from the creator of the "POSE" running method, Romanian Dr. Nicholas Romanov. One of the unexpected and pleasantly surprising things I did was to go to New Jersey and take a workshop with Shaun T in which there were only ten of us, which was the ultimate learning experience. He is almost like a rock star now.

Many of these fitness gurus I visited were so accomplished that it seemed like they had hit the ground running. I began to regard the slower pace of my own fitness career with some disappointment. But then I stoppped to consider the agave plant. Did you know the Americana agave plant takes ten years to bloom? And that the Kurinji Plant takes twelve years to bloom? The Madagascar Palm takes 100 years to bloom! I never started competing in fitness until I was thirty-eight and in Spartan Races at age fifty-three. I started slow, I was what they call a late bloomer. I am saying that because it isn't when you start that matters, it's about getting started.

No matter what your goals are, give yourself the time it takes to develop, blossom, and grow. When I decided to compete I had no formal training, only desire. I didn't have dance, gymnastics, modeling, or performance skills. I had only desire. I believe desire can take you to your destiny as long as you have determination.

After watching competitors that must've started when they were young, I realized I was not in their league, so I had to give myself time and opportunity to develop and grow. I decided to set a goal of competing in fitness until I was fifty. It was not until I reached my fifties that I placed in the top five not once, but five times at Fitness America. I began doing Reebok Spartan Races at age fifty-three, placing first in my age group twice and achieved my Spartan

Trifecta Medal after completing three Reebok Spartan races in four months' time—The Beast, Super, and Sprint.

Yes, you may start slow. Yes, you may lose a few times, but it takes guts, attitude, and belief in yourself and your ability to push forward. Win or lose, you will be okay. It's playing the game, getting involved, and going for it that will bring you success. You will bloom in time from all of the effort and hard work you put in. The sky is the limit. What I have found is that with passion and hard work, you can achieve almost anything.

I have had an amazing fitness career that just keeps evolving regardless of my age. When I started, I didn't realize you could make an income doing something so great and amazing like helping people get fit. When I left my abusive husband and had two small children to raise, I had to make a decision whether I wanted to follow my passion and make a living in fitness or pursue something more lucrative. I chose fitness. I believed, and still do, that doing what I love isn't like a job and that because of that, I'd be successful at it. "If you love what you do, you'll never work a day in your life!" There weren't very many people making a living in the fitness industry back then. When I took my first personal training certification, I thought, "Maybe I'll use this someday!" Fitness has been my passion ever since. I could have done many other things with more earning potential, but this has been my passion. I have stuck with it and it has stuck with me. Through thick and thin, ups and downs, highs and lows, fitness has been my mainstay, my rock, my go to. Fitness has been my outlet, my outreach, my way of helping myself and of helping others to be strong and courageous and to go after their dreams.

I began writing when someone suggested that I write an article about older competitors competing against younger ones. I said, "I'm not a writer." Famous last words. After pondering it a while, I thought, "I'll take a stab at it. What's the worst that can happen?" So I began writing a letter to the owner of Ms. Fitness contests and magazine. That letter was my first article. Soon after that, I began writing my own magazine column ("Fit over 40") for *Ms. Fitness* magazine, cover stories, and collaborated on a book. I found that I loved writing because it gave me a voice and a way of reaching out to others. When I was young, starry eyed and full of dreams, I never envisioned that at some point I would have my own brand, be the owner of a fitness studio, and be an established author to boot. When I was working out at home, snowed-in with two small children in Minot, North Dakota, I never dreamed that at some point I would be invited to work on the fitness portion of a book. I certainly never dreamed that it would be like a sequel to the *Fat Flush Fitness Plan* Joanie Greggains had written. I had the prestigious honor of collaborating on the fitness portion of *Fat Flush for Life* with best-selling author, Ann Louise Gittleman and now, I am the author of *The Sisterhood of S.W.E.A.T.*

1
Healthy Mind, Healthy Heart

Invest In You

Do your friends and loved ones enable you or do they empower you?

As a woman, I've noticed that many of us enjoy doing things in groups or with our friends, but there may come a time when you are trying to achieve greatness and reach goals that you have to ask yourself, "Are my friends setting me back or are they pushing me forward? Did I stay home from that workout because my friend did not go? Did I decide not to do that 10k because my friend that I always go with isn't going this year? Did I squelch my light because it was shining too brightly, making my friend feel less?" Sometimes friends, spouses, or family members don't push you forward because it makes them feel threatened. I've seen this stop many women in their tracks. Women take on the "mommy guilt" meaning they think, "I'm not cooking enough, I'm not home enough, I'm not doing enough," but the truth is that you're doing more than enough. It is okay to have something for yourself. It is a good example for your children to see you living and being your authentic self. Other sources of guilt could be called "wife guilt," (I need to spend more time with my spouse, I need to fix dinner for my spouse, etc.) or "breadwinner guilt," (I don't have time, I have so much work to do, etc.). Make fitness and wellbeing your top priority, not the lowest priority after you have met the needs of everyone else.

It's okay for your family to recognize that you have needs. Yes, your family and friends do need to feel your love and support but shouldn't you expect to receive the same from them? What your family needs most is a happy you. Ask yourself, "What am I not doing that I used to do, that I loved doing, and why?" You deserve to be excited when your feet hit the floor in the morning about what the day will bring. If you don't stay strong, how can you help someone else? If you're not empowered, how can you empower others? If you don't take care of yourself, how are you supposed to take care of someone else? Do you find yourself taking mere crumbs and eating burnt toast while everyone else eats biscuits? One of the biggest problems women face is being able to give themselves permission to invest in themselves. More often than not women may feel selfish when they take time away from family activities for themselves. There is no need to justify investing in you. Wanting something for you is reason enough. You do not need anyone else's permission to take care of and nurture yourself - that is your God given right. As women, we are usually the nurturers but we also need to refuel our tanks so that we have something to give. It is good for our children and spouses/partners to recognize that we, too, have needs. At the end of the day, when we invest in ourselves, we are going to be happier and will have more to give back to our loved ones. The only permission you need to live in your greatness is your own. Know your value and recognize your worth.

If you're not moving forward, you're moving backward. If you're not moving toward something, you're moving away from it.

"Every day, we make a choice to move toward what we want or further away. Choosing nothing is still making a choice."
-Lindaluation

Social Shaming

Be careful what you say to yourself because yours is the voice you listen to the most. What story are you telling yourself over and over in your head that you can't do, be, or have? Sometimes the stories we tell ourselves aren't even started by us. Somebody told us something about ourselves and we believed it.

We are more than our bodies. We need to step away from accepting the judgments we perceive through the media and by the court of public opinion to be fact. Recently in the media, Serena Williams' body image was criticized at the Grand Slam Chase for its muscularity and what they considered a lack of femininity. What? It's not feminine to be strong? In no way should Serena Williams, one of the world's most famous tennis players, be judged and shamed because she has a fit, muscular body. One would think that in the world of professional sports, an athlete would be praised and celebrated for her strength and power. On the other hand, neither should Kelly Clarkson be publicly shamed by the media for having a post baby body. Her body just performed one of life's greatest miracles. If I'm a swimsuit model, gorgeous, sexy and in touch with my sexuality, I shouldn't be judged and shunned by other women either. With this kind of attack, it's no surprise that women everywhere have body image issues. This will continue until we, as women, stand up and begin a discussion about it.

Be who you are! Let it shine unshackled, untamed, and unashamed. If you are an athlete, dancer, singer, teacher, brainiac, or mom, be that and be proud. Support other women. Instead of tearing each other down, build each other up. Help yourself and others rise to their fullest potential and greatest strength. We were not created to be the same so let's celebrate each other's differences. Developing a community of women celebrating other women is my greatest aspiration, dream, and hope. I believe that letting go of bitterness, jealousy, insecurities, the feeling that we are not good enough, and freeing ourselves from the belief that we can never be what we want to be will teach us to better support one another. When we are hard on others it is generally because we are hardest on ourselves. When we are gentler and kinder to ourselves it will enable us to celebrate other women because we are celebrating ourselves.

"Perfectionism crushes creativity—one of the most effective ways to start recovering from perfectionism is to start creating."
-Brené Brown.

Serena Williams said, "I just don't have time to be brought down. I have too many things to do, you know. I have Grand Slams to win. I have people to inspire. And that's what I'm here for." I think we should all have this mentality and be out there living our greatest lives with no time for living small.

I do not believe in shaming somebody because of their size or physical condition. I believe in love, acceptance, and encouragement. You may understand what fat shaming is, but there is also something called fit shaming. Fit shaming is the opposite of fat shaming and it occurs when someone is very envious of the person who lives a healthy and fit lifestyle and they try to shame them for it. Here is the bottom line: shaming of any kind is destructive behavior. It tears down the "shamer" as well as the "target." So the antidote to shaming is encouragement. I believe we should all be "encouragers."

As a woman, a health coach and a trainer, I do think that we should always do our very best job to take care of ourselves. That being said, I don't believe in eating a lot of junk or doing things that are self-sabotaging or that make me feel bad about myself. I don't believe in giving food that power. A very famous radio host was recently talking about how Kelly Clarkson needed to push away the deep dish pizza. Was Kelly Clarkson even eating deep dish pizza? The assumption as well as the judgment and shaming are inappropriate. I don't think we should judge each other but I do think we should educate one another.

Everybody should stay off the deep dish pizza. As a trainer, I find that deep dish pizza is one of the worst foods that anyone can eat. It can cause weight gain almost automatically because of the combination of white flour, fat and carbohydrates. The cheese alone causes dopamine to release in your brain and sets off comfort signals like a drug. Pizza enters your bloodstream like sugar and spikes insulin levels which, in turn, can result in weight gain and stored fat. Pizza is most likely to trigger cravings because it's loaded with fat, sugar, salt and dairy. I know that at the end of the day I feel better when I eat better, when I make more powerful choices. When I eat like crap, I feel like crap. If I eat too much ice cream and drink too much wine, I feel bloated.

At the end of the day, it's about learning how to enjoy good nutrition and occasional treats. I don't care what anyone says—if you're eating more than your fair share of junk, it isn't really going to make you feel very good long term. It might taste good going down, but that is just about it—instant gratification. The after effects of eating junk are not worth the pleasure of the taste. Health is wealth.

To each his own and to thine own self be true. If you don't want to work for something, then don't judge someone who does. For instance, I'm not an Olympic gymnast because I didn't spend hours in gymnastics but I have great respect and admiration for their developed skills and dedication. Another example—if I like to eat ice cream, cake, candy and pizza, I want that and I enjoy that. I may look great but I shouldn't expect to have a "six pack" set of abs. A six pack comes with discipline and diet. So I shouldn't judge someone who wants six pack abs and who puts in the work to have them. Nor should they judge me if I choose to eat chocolate.

As you begin your journey towards a healthier lifestyle, it may surprise some of you to know that not everyone is going to support your new choices. You may be ridiculed, made fun of, and even be peer pressured to veer off track.

When you begin going after your dreams and making big changes for the better, people tend to lash out because your choices make them uncomfortable. The criticism may come from unexpected sources like family and friends at the least opportune times. Sometimes the grief people give you will really make you begin to question yourself and think about dimming your light. Here's a phrase you may want to remember during those times: "I don't eat [fill in the blank]." It requires no explanation and no excuses; it's just a simple statement. "No, thank you, I don't eat pizza. But I'll enjoy a salad with you!"

I know we really hate to be different and stand out. There is nothing like having a whole crowd of people stare at you when you whip out your container of tuna and broccoli at a social function. The social pressure can be so intense that you feel the need to be like everyone else just because you don't want to stand out. The questions and excuses will begin flooding your brain—"Can't I just go off plan this weekend because I'm going on a camping trip?" "Oh, my friends want to go out tonight," or, "I have a wedding and I think I will have to start tomorrow."

If you want to see a change, you have to make a change. Stop the celebratory eating at every occasion and start celebrating your health by honoring your body and filling it with fresh, good food. I know we hate to be different and stand out, but having the body of your dreams requires planning, discipline, and some cajones. Sometimes you've just got to dig deep and reach down into that place inside of yourself and find your courage. The kind of courage as in Lord of the Rings when Gandalf says, and my favorite line to date, "You shall not pass." That's the steely, determined grit it takes to withstand any storm and to come out riding the waves like you were born to do so.

When women are ballsy, they are considered bitchy while men are considered strong. I consider them brave.

People will never admit that they admire or envy you. Instead of working hard enough to achieve what you have, they may say and do things to try and bring you down to their level. It is really important to recognize this for what it is and to surround yourself with positive people who support you. Sometimes you can't fit into a round hole because you're a square peg. Don't ever let somebody make you feel bad about being a square peg because square pegs rock. Sometimes, for greatness to happen, you have to go through hardships to clear the way for yourself. If you have haters around then you've got to get them out of your way to arrive at your greatest success and purpose.

If people are talking about you, you must be doing something that is shaking up their world a bit, kind of like shining a flashlight in the dark and it's making them realize where they are lacking in their own lives. They can either rise to the challenge you've presented by your living, breathing example or talk about you and to try to bring you down. You must also realize that when it seems someone hates on you for your new lifestyle or transformation, most often they internally hate upon themselves. This is your opportunity to encourage them to join your journey. One of my favorite quotes is: "A light shines brightest in the dark." So shine on!

"To avoid criticism, say nothing, do nothing, have nothing."
~Aristotle

Eating to Fit in

Does any of the following sound familiar?

- I have to eat it because it's what's being served.
- We are going out with our friends to a greasy foods sports bar. There is no way I can eat healthy.
- It's the holidays! I couldn't possibly eat healthy.
- I know it's a heart attack walking but my grandmother baked it for me.
- I like to snack during my favorite shows.
- We are going to a sports tournament where everyone will be eating pizza, hot dogs, popcorn, candy, chips, and soda. I'll stand out like a sore thumb.
- In social situations, I feel like I might alienate other women and make them feel less if I'm eating perfectly and they are not.

Set the pace, be the trendsetter, bring your own healthy dish, and look at the menu in advance. Stop eating for entertainment or to fit in. Decide your plan of action in advance. You can eat healthy or you can eat guilty. The next time you are faced with a social situation, try choosing mouthwatering healthy food that is cooked just right. You may choose to eat your healthy food before you go so that you do not have to consume quantities of food that you know you really don't want to eat. You will feel so good about yourself that the feeling of deprivation for not having those ooey-gooey cheese fries will fade.

Get used to asking for what you want.

At the Restaurant -

Learning how to order is the key:

- "I'll take my chicken grilled without any added oils."
- "In addition, may I have a double order of steamed broccoli instead of the mashed potatoes and white rice please?"
- "I would like my salad with romaine lettuce, onions, mushrooms, and apples, minus the croutons and cheese, thank you."
- "Also, if you would, bring my dressing of oil and vinegar on the side."
- "Please take the white sauce off of my chicken." ("I'm lactose intolerant" always works. They don't need to know that you are just really intolerant to the extra 500 calories that are probably in the sauce.)
- "Sorry, no bread for me. I don't do gluten." (No one needs to know you don't do gluten because it makes you feel tired, bloated, and puffy.)

With Friends -

- When they start passing the alcohol around: "I only drink hi-octane cocktails. I'll have cranberry juice please."
- Bring your own healthy dish.
- With grandma, try the two bite rule or plan it as treat meal.
- Choose the restaurant.

Special Occasion/Holiday Eating Tips

(Every day is special occasion to celebrate your life.)

1. Don't go to any party hungry. Eat a salad beforehand to keep yourself from overeating holiday goodies.
2. The yummy chocolate meringue mousse with a cherry on top may very well taste lighter than air, but it is probably laden with too many unhealthy fats, sodium, and sugar. Count calories because they do matter and will show up on your person somewhere.

3. Beware of holiday beverages. They will, without a doubt, add inches to your waistline. Drink water, coffee or tea instead, which will fill you up and has zero calories.
4. Drink some hot tea or have a cup of soup before your next holiday gathering. Studies show that having some hot soup or tea before a meal can decrease hunger, increase fullness, and reduce one's overall calorie consumption.
5. Plan ahead. Bring your own healthy treat to the next party you attend. Chances are others will be thankful because they are trying to watch their waistlines too.
6. Don't skip exercise. Remain consistent throughout the holidays with your exercise regimen to keep holiday weight gain to a minimum.
7. During holiday/special occasion gatherings, play games, dance and be active. Make fun the focus instead of food.
8. Follow the 90-10 rule. Eat great 90% of the time and save the other 10% for a special occasion indulgence.

2
Define Your Path

Are You on a Journey or a Mission?

I was out running the track early one morning with my boot camp group and some guy asked me, "What did you have for breakfast?" I thought for a second and said, "I had motivation for breakfast." That's what you have when you set goals. You get out of bed in the morning because you have a reason that is strong enough to make you get up, put your shoes on, and hit the track at 6am.

Are you on a journey or a mission? There is nothing wrong with being on either one, but it's good to be clear about which one you're on!

When you are on a journey, you don't know where you're headed and you are unsure of where you'll end up. You may get blown around by the wind and feel like you are bouncing around like a ping pong ball. It's sort of like when you decide one week that you want to lose thirty pounds and that you're going to work out every day, faithfully. Or, because of the time crunch, you become a weekend warrior instead. The work week starts and almost immediately, you get sucked into the swamp of your life. You only get to work out two days, stop, and not start again until the end of the month. This can be very frustrating. Things have to stop being all or nothing or they will soon be nothing. Exercise is an appointment you make with yourself, plan into your schedule, and keep.

19

The mentality that it has to be hours upon hours of exercise to be effective is hogwash. This is the story we tell ourselves over and over. It's so untrue.

One of the primary reasons people discontinue their exercise regimen is simply a lack of motivation. They start out all gung-ho, usually because something inspired them, but all too soon, they begin to fizzle out. Inspiration isn't long lasting enough to get them to their destination. In fact, without a strong set of reasons to achieve one's goals, people more often than not will give in to the temptation to quit. Without a powerful reason "why" in front of us, it is easy to get distracted by everyday life and lose focus. When you find your WHY, you are on a mission, you know what you want and everything you do has purpose and a set intention! Your mind is set on what you want to accomplish and you set plans in motion to accomplish your mission. You have a detailed plan and are 100 % committed to backing that up with action. You will move Heaven and Earth to reach your goal. You have calculated the risks and the cost to reaching your end goal. You can't rest until your mission is accomplished and will do whatever it takes to reach your objective—whether it is to run the extra mile, or swim the ocean, or eat that yucky butternut squash your trainer is always pushing on you. A mission moves and drives you to do the things that will take you to completion. I'm pretty sure I know some famous athletes that would amputate a body part if it meant achieving their goal. They are definitely on a mission. A mission is what it takes. With a mission, there is more of a sense of urgency. On a journey, you are unsure yet of how to get where you're going. A journey is more about the experience of traveling from one destination to the next. Many of us are focused so much on the destination we forget to enjoy the journey. John Steinbeck described the journey when he said, "A journey is like marriage. The certain way to be wrong is to think you control it."

My philosophy is that you are almost always on a journey so you might as well enjoy it. I think it's important to have both! I'm enjoying my journey more because I'm on a mission. My mission is to help women to love themselves when they look in the mirror and to have the ability to transfer that love into supporting one another.

Give Yourself a Pass to Suck until You Don't

Slow and steady gets results. Scenario: Two people start exercising together. One says to the other, "OMG, I can't keep up with this. It's too hard, everyone is leaving me behind, and besides, I'm old and overweight." The other says, "Well, I know if I keep this up I am going to get in better shape. I want this so bad that I am not going to give up." The first person ducks out of class and never comes back. The second person loses twenty-five pounds in ten weeks.

I see this time and time again. People come to class or start an exercise regimen while being so worried about what everyone else is doing and whether they are keeping up or not with the twenty-five year old doing 100 reps at the speed of light. My advice to them is that slow and steady wins the race. Don't blow yourself out. Don't worry about what everyone else is doing; you will get there in your own time. Focus only on what you can do today, then tomorrow it will be more and, before you know it, peeps will be having trouble keeping up with you. Now don't get me wrong, good old competition can be a great thing when you use it to help make you better or to push yourself harder. But this may not be the best thing to do during the first week or the first month of taking classes. This may be contrary to what most people believe when they begin a boot camp class or any type of exercise regimen, but you don't have to be the best or work out the hardest to get great results!

So many times when people don't give their all and do what the plan says 100%, they think they may as well do nothing. The thinking becomes they've failed so they may as well quit. Give yourself a pass to suck until you don't. I want this to be your mantra. Say it over and over to yourself. If this remotely resembles the attempts you've made in the past, why not try starting out with 70% of whatever exercise plan you start? Then, as you get used to it and get it down, maybe you'll do 80%. The end goal in mind will be 90/10. Do 90% of your plan perfectly and allow yourself a 10% error margin. The 10% is a weekly treat meal, a day off, running two miles instead of three, or time to relax. The people who usually get the most results are the quiet, determined ones who put forth consistent effort and never quit.

Motivation = Transformation

A lack of motivation is really just the lack of a powerful purpose in front of you. Yes, exercise is a science, but it doesn't matter how scientific you get about it if you don't get up and put it to use. Here are some tips on motivation:

How to Stay Motivated

1. Set some goals and write them down.

    Discipline is remembering what you want. When you get out of bed each morning, remind yourself why exercise is important to achieving your goals. Constantly reminding yourself of your goals will keep you focused.

    "Without goals, and plans to reach them, you are like a ship that has set sail with no destination." ~Fitzhugh Dodson

2. Make a commitment to yourself to exercise even when you don't necessarily feel like it.

    Commitment is follow through even when the initial excitement has faded. Even if you don't feel like it, just get into your workout gear and head for the gym. Take one step at a time and soon it will become a routine.

    "Desire is the key to motivation, but it's determination and commitment to an unrelenting pursuit of your goal - a commitment to excellence - that will enable you to attain the success you seek." ~Mario Andretti

3. Allow flexibility in your exercise regimen.

    Avoid all or nothing mentality. When it comes to exercise, do what works for you and fits into your lifestyle. One day missed isn't failure. If you set the bar too high, you might give up before you even get started.

    "The greatest barrier to success is the fear of failure." ~Sven Goran Eriksson

4. Benchmark your progress.

    Take photos every four weeks, have a professional measure your body fat composition, or weigh and measure. Visually seeing the difference will go a long way in helping you stay on track.

    "Obstacles are those frightful things you see when you take your eyes off your goal." ~Henry Ford

5. Make a list of all the benefits of exercise.

    Exercise boosts brain power, you will enjoy better sleep, increases stamina, wards off illnesses, elevates your mood, provides stress relief, improves the cardiovascular system, provides you with more energy, raises endorphin levels, helps weight loss, strengthens muscles, builds self-esteem and confidence, fosters creativity, and the list goes on.

    "Movement is a medicine for creating change in a person's physical, emotional, and mental states." ~Carol Welch

6. Be accountable to someone.

    Hire a trainer, recruit an exercise buddy, join a gym, or participate in a group fitness class. Accountability—knowing that someone is waiting for you to exercise with them—can be great motivation not to miss a workout.

    "Accountability breeds response-ability." ~Stephen R. Covey

7. Make it fun!

    If you are dreading your exercise plan, pick a mode of exercise that you enjoy so you will actually look forward to it. Exercise should feel like a recess. Those who enjoy exercise will be much more consistent.

    "People rarely succeed unless they have fun in what they are doing." ~Dale Carnegie

8. Subscribe to a fitness publication.

    Various fitness magazines contain success stories as well as the latest exercise research. They even have tips on how to perfect your exercise techniques. This can serve as a constant source of inspiration as well as information.

    "The best effect of any book is that it excites the reader to self-activity."
    ~Thomas Carlyle

9. Reward yourself often and pat yourself on the back for every goal achieved.

    Reward yourself with something other than food. At the end of your workout, try taking a hot bath and soaking for an extra ten minutes. Plan something fun at the end of every exercise week such as a massage, a fun shopping trip, a spa day, a movie, or even catch up on your reading while sitting in front of the fire.

    "This I do know beyond any reasonable doubt. Regardless of what you are doing, if you pump long enough, hard enough and enthusiastically enough, sooner or later the effort will bring forth the reward." ~Zig Ziglar

10. Keep your workouts fresh and prevent them from becoming stale and boring.

    Change your workout routine every 4-6 weeks and try something new. Doing something new can keep you motivated and on track. Mixing things up a bit will make your workouts seem shorter and more interesting.

    "Insanity: doing the same thing over and over again and expecting different results." ~Albert Einstein

11. Visualize yourself the way you want to be.

    Top athletes use this technique to achieve greatness. When you can visualize yourself achieving your dreams, chances are you will. What you believe, you will achieve.

"If you want to reach a goal, you must 'see the reaching' in your own mind before you actually arrive at your goal." ~Zig Ziglar

12. Journal your progress.

   The simple act of writing it down will make your weight loss efforts 50% more successful according to a recent study from Kaiser Permanente's Center for Health.

   "The Journey is the reward." ~ancient Chinese proverb

13. Sign up for a 10K or a marathon.

   This can be a great motivation to exercise on a regular basis. Before you know it, with regular training, you will be in great shape.

   "Set your goals high and don't stop until you get there." ~Bo Jackson

14. Schedule your exercise time just like an appointment.

   Make it a top priority and you will reap the many benefits that regular exercise provides.

   "The key is not to prioritize what's on your schedule, but to schedule your priorities." ~Steven R. Covey

15. Download your favorite tunes on your iPod.

   A recent study conducted out of Brunel University's School of Sport and Education by researcher Dr. Costas Karageorghis suggests that listening to upbeat music will motivate you to exercise harder and increase your endurance by 15%. The theory is that listening to music elevates our mood and erases some of the pain we would normally feel during training which allows us to go the distance.

   "Take a music bath once or twice a week for a few seasons. You will find it is to the soul what a water bath is to the body." ~Oliver Wendell Holmes

Setting goals and having some way to measure your success is the catalyst for anyone who wants to see results. Let's face it, seeing results is what keep us motivated.

3
Building Confidence to Build Health

You Are Good Enough

Why compare when you can have confidence instead?

I've been in the fitness business for thirty-two years now. Over that span I've dabbled a little bit in everything from personal training to coordinating group fitness programs to writing for fitness publications. Currently, I've settled into running my own fitness organization specifically devoted to fulfilling the needs of women. After spending years of time with women from all walks of life, I have come to the conclusion that the way you see yourself is very important. Recently, on one of my women's boot camp retreats, a very dear friend of mine was picking herself apart; she just couldn't see herself as beautiful. (She is one of the sweetest and most beautiful women I know.)

It was then that it really hit home for me how many women think they will become beautiful once they lose weight, have plastic surgery, or buy a new wardrobe. They think that once they arrive at that perfect place that all will be right with the world, but that perfect place never comes. Confidence and beauty cannot be bought no matter how much money you spend on fillers, Botox, facelifts, boob jobs, and liposuction. It will never be enough unless you spend some time finding out who you are and begin working on the inside.

You see, if you don't believe you're beautiful, it doesn't matter how many beauty regimens you subscribe to or how often you work out. True beauty and confidence come from within. Beauty truly begins when we free ourselves from perfectionism and accept ourselves the way we are. We are already beautiful, all we need to do is reach out and claim it.

We are so much more than just the way we look. We are all special in our own unique ways. When we focus on our flaws that is all we will see. Highlighting our differences and following our passions is what makes us stand out as individuals. In other words, just be happy with yourself because you are perfect just as you are. Now, I am not saying you should not strive to achieve more or become better. I am saying you should try to be a better "YOU" and not a lesser version of someone else. Embrace where you are. Like Judy Garland said, "Always be a first rate version of yourself, instead of a second rate version of somebody else." Judy learned early on what it was like to be compared to others and felt like she needed to fit into a certain criteria. She tried to fit into the Hollywood mold. But Judy Garland was one of the greatest stars of our time because she didn't fit the mold; she wasn't a carbon copy of everyone else. That is why she stood out. Judy was unique, ageless, and timeless. She learned to be a first rate version of herself. I believe a lot of times, as women, we are told what we're supposed to be like and try to gear ourselves to a certain image that the media has portrayed as the perfect woman. When you evaluate your worth by others' opinions, you will always be losing.

As Theodore Roosevelt once said, "Comparison truly is the thief of joy." God has made us unique and individual. No fingerprints or DNA are the same. We all have something unique to bring to the table. When we are living our passion and purpose we are all beautiful. The more you love yourself the less you hate on other people. If you're insecure about yourself, you're automatically going to be more critical of others. When you are critical of others, you're going to naturally be more critical of yourself. Break the vicious cycle by taking action steps to become confident and happier with yourself and you will automatically create an environment that breeds confidence.

One thing I learned through fitness pageants and competing the hard way is not to compare yourself to others. Just because a judge or pageant picks another girl doesn't mean you're not great. Just because that girl came out on top doesn't mean that she is better than you. You're both great in your own unique ways. Maybe the judge prefers strawberry instead of raspberry. Instead of saying raspberry must be a crappy flavor, recognize that it's not about worth, rather it's about preference. Realize that something bigger is at stake than a trophy or winning a contest. You've set yourself up to get validation from an external source and have given up your power. Take your power back! Celebrate yourself and realize that someone out there is bound to like your flavor because it's a great flavor. There is really nothing to be gained by trying to live up to other people's expectations. Live in celebration of who you are, step away from the crowd, and let your true self shine through.

Have you ever noticed the way certain people walk into a room and every head turns. I call that the "IT FACTOR." In the looks department, these individuals may just be a little bit above average or even by aesthetic standards nothing special, but they just exude confidence. The "It Factor" comes from being your authentic self, unapologetically, unabashedly, just knowing who you are, and making no apologies for it. God doesn't make junk. If anyone makes you feel bad about being yourself, maybe it is time to distance yourself from that person.

If you're not a confident person now and you find yourself constantly comparing yourself to others and feeling that you don't measure up, try these strategies:

1. Focus on being the best possible version of yourself because everyone else is taken.

    We all have flaws but we also all have strengths. Winners focus on their strengths and don't beat themselves up for their shortcomings.

2. Set goals that make you stretch.

    If your goals don't scare you they're probably not big enough. The good fruit on the tree is out on the limb. Climb out of your comfort zone and eat that juicy red apple.

3. Celebrate your successes. Don't wait for someone else's permission or affirmation.

   Applaud every step you make for the positive. Celebrate yourself. Don't wait for others to validate you.

4. Practice gratitude for the greatness you have within and enjoy and celebrate the greatness in others.

   The law of abundance says that there is enough to go around. The law of deprivation says that if you have *this*, that means there is less for others. Life is better when you view your glass as half full.

"Envy destroys, gratitude enjoys."
~Lindaluation

5. Here is one of my favorites and one that my husband, Tracy, says to me constantly: Focus on what you can control.

   When we worry, we are giving in to fear instead of having faith. Worry only grows warts.

"Comparing your journey to someone else's is a good way to miss out on the journey you are actually on." ~Jon Acuff

Maybe your journey is to be a coach, a competitor, a teacher, a leader, a follower, a doer, a builder, a believer, a writer, a reader, an engineer, a playwright, a director, a photographer, etc. If you're so busy comparing yourself to others then you may miss the journey you're actually supposed to be on.

I am feeling great writing this because I know that beyond a shadow of a doubt that this is my purpose, it's what I'm called to do. I feel excited, alive, and full of endless possibilities. I want you to think back to the last time you felt like that. What makes you feel like that? Honor yourself and do more of what makes you feel excited to get out of bed in the morning. I want you so in your purpose that when your feet touch the floor in the morning, you're so excited you can hardly wait for the day to begin.

I believe each and every one of us has a significant purpose so stop trying to fit into a round hole when you're a square peg. Society tries to make women think they're supposed to be a certain way, most of which makes us feel as if we can never measure up. Stop the madness; give no one that much power over you. Revel in who you are.

If others aren't bashing us, we may be bashing ourselves. We can be our own worst critics. Self-bashing - your voice is the one you listen to the most so it's really important what you say to yourself. Be your own best friend. The spoken word is powerful. Speak energy and life and positivity into your existence. We are amazing and unique. We can grow. We can change. We don't have to be who we were yesterday. We can evolve. We can be who we want to be today. Don't look back, look forward to the future because the best is yet to come.

"Be willing to let go of who you think you should be
in order to be who you are." ~Brené Brown

I can remember going to a yoga conference where the exercise was to hold up your arm and clench your hand as tight as you could, making a fist, then resist while the opposing party tried to push it down. The first time you are supposed to have a negative thought, think skeptically while being strong. I resisted as hard as I could but, guess what, my opponent was able to push my arm down. The second time I was supposed to think of a positive thought while my partner pushed as hard as she could, and she could not push my arm down. This simple exercise really proved to me the power of a negative thought versus a positive one and how we should focus on the positive.

We can choose how we want to think about things. The way we think about things really influences how things turn out. People can go through the same experience and come out on top or come out in the dump. Really what it all boils down to is attitude. I really believe attitude is 90% of everything.

I still remember having a participant that had come to my boot camp for a six week special offer. This one particular day I had what I like to call the "super humans" in my class—personal trainers, boot camp instructors, competitors— and I sent them out on a run as their warm-up. During the warm-up, the special offer participant talked to another gal that had been coming for a short while and said, "Don't you find this discouraging? I can't even keep up with these people. They all are in such great shape. I might as well give up and quit." The other gal said, "I'm not worried about anyone else. I'm just here to get in shape." She started out always being the last one back from the run, from the lunges, the burpee's, the box jumps, but she just put one foot in front of the other and continued on, not comparing herself to others. I led her all the way through losing over seventy pounds and entering a fitness competition and man, she was ripped with a six pack. There are several things I want you to get out of this story. First, you never know where you might end up. You've just got to put one foot in front of the other and get started. Second, don't compare yourself to others. And last, the one who quit and walked out because she didn't believe she could ever achieve what these other people had achieved, because she expected to be where the "super humans" were at and it was too early in the game, she didn't give herself a chance to develop and grow. So, truly, it's all in the way you look at things.

Move away from perfection. Be happy with yourself right now, in this very moment. Your best is the best you can do. Don't throw out the baby with the bathwater when you end up making a less desirable choice. Dust yourself off and pick yourself up, realizing it is the majority of your choices that matter, not a moment of weakness.

Girl on Girl Crime

This is something so relevant yet so potent that nobody wants to talk about it for fear they may create some "girl on girl crime." That's right, you got it, girl drama. Chances are high that if you are a woman, at some point, you are going to be the victim of some type of girl drama. Here's the scenario: Two girls are BFF's but all the sudden they are not speaking because they had a significant difference of opinion. One will talk about the other and try to get their mutual friends and family to choose sides. If you are the mutual friend of the two BFF's, try to remember in any disagreement that there are always two sides to the story. Dr. Phil always says, "No matter how flat you smash a pancake there's always two sides." Stay out of the hornet's nest by refusing to choose sides or participate in petty gossip. When you judge someone based on hearsay or what you think happened, you are not only cheating them but you are cheating yourself as well. Help put the fire out by choosing not to participate. If you are the one involved in the BFF dispute, keep your dignity and act with integrity, this says a lot about you. Here's the thing—trying to destroy each other benefits nobody. When we hate someone, we are giving them power over us. Trust me, you may go through hell at first because, ladies, let's face it, when we are aggravated, hurt, angry or upset, we can be formidable. The temptation will be to strike back or play the "he-said-she-said game." The further away you get, you're going to realize you take your power back by avoiding negativity. Don't get drawn into that. Take the high road and change your focus to what really matters. Unfortunately, girl drama is a game you can't win. Diffuse drama and gossip by refusing to feed it or give it the time of day. When someone comes to you, talking about your friend or mutual acquaintance, remember in the words of my Papaw, "If they talk about Sue, they will probably talk about you." Put some time back in your day by avoiding girlfriend drama because it's a time sucker. It isn't always easy and it isn't always pretty, but in the end, it's worth avoiding.

Some people will try to take advantage of you. That's why it's up to you to be the gatekeeper of your life. Not everyone belongs in your life, at least not in a front row seat. The following types of people have made the honorable mention list.

Carrie Copycat - She wants to be you, but I'm pretty sure there is only one you. Sorry, this space is taken. There is only one original.

Negative Nelly - She will point out why everything you want to do is wrong and how you can't possibly do it.

Debbie Downer - Takes the fun out of everything. She just brings the positive mood of the room down.

Envious Eve - She will copy everything you do. Everything you have soon becomes hers, including your friends. She will suck the life right out of you if you let her. Be careful with this one. When you try to separate yourself from her, she may try to bring you down. They even made a movie about this one called *All About Eve* starring Bette Davis.

Tina Two-Faced - She likes to play both sides of the fence because she's only interested in what's in it for her. Only give her the information you want her to have. She will talk about you behind your back and only get the story half right.

Hannah Half-Truth - She twists the truth every which way but loose. She majors in half-truths and twists the rest to suit herself or gain the sympathy of others.

Tootsie Taker - All she ever does is take from you and others. She takes your ideas, knowledge, money, reputation, and spirit if you let her. She is all about herself and what you can do for her. She thinks that what is yours should be hers and she will use you as a stepping stone to get it. If you're a giver, this personality type can be toxic for you. Ask yourself what are she is bringing to the table—is it mutually beneficial? You've already given her enough, you don't need to give her your peace of mind too.

Maxine the Manipulator - When you say, "No," she may begin to bully you, try to make you feel guilty, then start to beg, and maybe even cry. If this doesn't work, look out. She will try to come at you with threats. The manipulator only wants her own way. She is arrogant and thinks she is above accountability. She plays the victim card really well.

Ursula the One-Upper - Whatever you do, she has to one-up you or do you one better. You went on vacation and did speed boating while she cruised the Pacific in a yacht. The movie *Bride Wars* with Kate Hudson and Anne Hathaway is a perfect example of one-upmanship at its finest.

Sally Superior - She constantly tries to bring you down so she can elevate herself. This stems from insecurities that she may have about herself. Though tedious, the reason this personality is a little easier to deal with is because trying to make others look bad to make herself look good tends to backfire.

Freedom is letting go of the court of public opinion. When you kick group B people to the curb, you automatically make room for group A people. The best thing to do when something is dragging you down and taking away your mojo is to set something in place that pushes you forward. Even if you're not feeling it, set a new goal, start taking steps towards that goal, and you'll be able to move away from the energy-sucking drama.

When you face these types of individuals, you may feel like quitting your mission because it zaps your energy and your motivation. It's not that you should quit anything, rather you may need to quit the person. The quote I am most reminded of is, "Just because you have a flat tire doesn't mean you go out and slash the rest of your tires." There are just some personalities you may need to separate yourself from. I call these toxic relationships. So maybe you did everything right and you still got screwed over. Try again. But if that doesn't work, don't be afraid to disconnect. The older I get, the more I realize that you only have so much energy so you need to spend it wisely. You won't have enough fuel to get where you're going if you waste it all on the negative. Negative energy drains you, positive energy fills you up. Having the wisdom to know the difference is a game changer.

Guard your energy. Take every rock thrown at you and build your house. You know who you are and it's not the mud that someone has thrown at you in the way of words or deeds. You are a morning glory, not a shrinking violet. Rise and SHINE your light brighter in case someone has mistaken who you are. Shining bright in the light of day, everything becomes crystal clear. Yes, you've taken a beating. Stand up and fight. Be you, be proud, and all of your actions will speak loud. Deep down, maybe you have fears that they are right about you. Well, check yourself girl, then move on. Be who you are, not who they say you are. Don't let self-doubt and fear of judgement hold you hostage.

Drama Facts:

A. Spending your precious time on drama is a waste of perfectly good energy.

B. The more time you spend with drama, the less time you spend working towards your purpose and living your dreams.

C. Every moment you unhook yourself from drama is a moment you save.

It's hard for people to hide when you shine a light on them, exposing them for who they truly are. Sometimes you've got to hold people's feet to the fire to know what's truly there. Be grateful when things like this happen and people like this leave, taking their drama with them. This will leave you more time to spend on the people you want to be around that treat you right.

Sometimes, when you have to make tough decisions or you're on your way to something good, you may be unfairly judged. It will hurt like hell. Rather than spending your time trying to diffuse unfair judgment and gossip, focus on building the new. The proof is in the pudding. The beauty of your life is it's a picture that you are painting, a masterpiece, and it is not finished until the last brush stroke has been laid down.

When you feel like you're being judged unfairly, focus your energy on positive things. You have no control over what others think of you or what others try to do to you. You only have control over yourself, the way you react, the way you respond, and the things that you forgive.

1.   Forgiveness is for you because it sets you free.

2.   Do some self-examination. Is it possible that you made a mistake or an error in judgment?

3.   Own your stuff and make amends if it's your bad.

4.   Ask yourself, "Who among us doesn't make mistakes?" We all do, it's human nature. Give yourself a pass to be human.

5.   Focus on what you can control.

As long as you're still stuck in the past you can't get on with your life. Every day is a new opportunity to walk away from the shoreline, to forge your dreams, to leave the past behind, to make things new again, to forgive, and to love. The great thing about life is that it is new every morning.

Don't let anyone steal the joy of your morning. Every morning is a new day and a new chance to get things right. Make sure not to let the seeds of bitterness take root, think about what kind of crop you want to grow. The seeds of bitterness can do so much damage, not just to the person you're upset with but to you. In the light of day, forgiveness is the key. You will realize that God had his hand on you the whole time. He led you through the storm to take you where you are going. A kite rises against the wind, not with it, so when you have a storm, be thankful because it's going to take you into your greatness if you let it. Your morning is so important. It sets the tone for your entire day. Value it and it will pay dividends.

*"When you hold onto your history, you do it at the
expense of your destiny."* ~Bishop Jakes

You are not your mistakes. Today may be a struggle just to push through because you feel so far away from where you were when there wasn't all of this drama in your life. You may not feel like doing your normal routine at first but just do a little and see how it goes. At first, you may not feel as strong as you were and quite frankly, it may suck, but once you start pushing through, you will remember who you are. You are not the disaster that has happened to you. You are not what is being said about you behind your back. You are not a bad person like you might be being made out to be. You are strong and you can move on. For whatever reason—your fault, their fault, or both people's fault— the relationship may have just stopped working. Don't waste time playing the blame game. You may have to bail on the relationship because it is unhealthy. It's not giving up. There is just no need to beat a dead horse and it's okay to admit when something just isn't working for you anymore. Sometimes you may have to clear the space to move on to start having success again.

Life Lessons:

- Hate is never the best option.
- You never get anywhere in life by tearing other people down.
- Never base your self-worth on somebody else's opinion.
- Push through to you.
- It's okay to pull the plug on something that's not working for you.
- One of the best ways to get over something is to start moving on.

Negative Energy Cleanse

- Does this thought bring me up or bring me down?
- Do my thoughts tear me or someone else down?
- Are my thoughts critical of myself or others?
- Is my thinking full of doubt or fear?
- Am I harboring resentment or holding grudges?

Positive Energy Builder:

- Are my thoughts confident and powerful?
- Is my thinking edifying, uplifting, and building me or someone else up?
- Forgive and move on.
- Let go and let life flow. (Relinquish the need to control.)
- Trust that life will work out the way it's supposed to.

Why dwell on negative thoughts when you can be thinking of all the moments that have made up your life that are worth cherishing and remembering? Memories I cherish are when my grandmother, Ruth, used to dry my hair by the fire, or when I planted a garden with my grandfather, Bert, and when the strawberries were ready for picking there were very few in my bucket because I was eating them all. Or the year my brother, Mark, gave me a gift because we were having a hard time making ends meet. He gave me $1,000 to pay on my mortgage. Or the time my son, Jake, left roses on my car, on the countertop, in the refrigerator and on the computer to let me know he thought I was special. Or the card my daughter, Tiffany, made me that said, "To the one who gives birth and has eyes in the back of her head." She is an artist so that explains the homemade cards and the blue food dye she squirted into my Easter bunny cake. Special, huh? Or my songwriter son, Michael, constantly serenading me in the kitchen with his precious gift of music. Or on my 50th birthday, when my husband, Tracy, went so out of his way to give me a birthday party that I will always cherish. Or the smell of my mother's homemade apple pie, made special, just for me. These are the memories that lift me up and in times of trouble remind me of who I am. My dad used to say, "There's enough positive things in this world to think about, think on those things." You can let your struggles take you down or bring you up. Grow from them, learn from them, and embrace the life lessons that they present to you.

> *"When you show deep empathy toward others, their defensive energy goes down, and positive energy replaces it. That's when you can get more creative in solving problems."* ~Stephen R. Covey

You can't run on empty.

Our society is running around tired, especially moms. More often than not, we find ourselves exhausted and running on fumes. When afternoon comes, we find that we've hit a wall and the majority of us wish we could lie down and take a nap, but we can't. Does this sound familiar?

Carve some space out for yourself. You're no good to anyone when you're run ragged. What would some breathing room look like to you? Perhaps it would include time for a cup of coffee, reading the paper, sleeping in, getting your hair done, or having the time to try out a new recipe and actually enjoying the cooking process because you're not overly stressed, rushed, or tired. Whatever you need to do in order to carve, find, and protect time for you, do it. Put you at the top of your to-do list. This will create space for your creative juices to flow, your productivity to soar, and will leave you feeling fulfilled. When saying yes to something, ask yourself, "Does this activity drain me or sustain me?"

Squeezing in me time is always worth it, even if it's just for a little bit. How are you going to be able to take care of everybody else if you don't take care of yourself? How are you going to have anything to give if you don't fill up your cup with some me time? Carving out some time and creating space for yourself is important to your overall frame of mind and creativity. Once you've created breathing space, you will be much more productive and energetic.

Three Energy Boosting Supplements:

Maca - helps to decrease menopausal symptoms, depression, and balances hormones. It can also increase libido, energy levels, athletic performance, muscle building, and bone density. Though Maca helps energy levels, it does not place added stress on the adrenals. It also supports thyroid health.

Ashwagandha - is an adaptogen with healing benefits that are great for stress, fatigue, and energy. It stabilizes blood sugar, helps to lower cholesterol, and improves memory and concentration.

Nutritional Yeast - Brewer's yeast has nutritional value and is not to be confused with the type of yeast that causes yeast infections and grows in your stomach and multiplies, robbing you of health benefits. This type of yeast is good for you. Nutritional yeast is a complete protein source, provides a significant amount of B12 (which really ramps up sustained energy levels throughout the day), is loaded with minerals, and is full of fiber. It has a very nutty, cheesy flavor and is great as a seasoning for your food.

My father, Herbert, used to make all sorts of healthy concoctions in the blender and stick out his tongue to show me the color. Very scientific. It was very dark green when he used wheat grass and bright cherry red when from his cranberry juice mixture. He was always excited to try anything that he thought was good for him. My father taught me to appreciate and respect my body and not to abuse it with chemicals or harsh drugs because it is wonderfully made. He used to go on about all the different chemical processes that the body goes through to function and how amazing that process truly is. He impressed upon me how we didn't want to mess with that process. Now, years later, here I am doing the same thing.

My Energy Boosting, Liver Cleaning Concoction:
(Drink first thing in the morning for best results.)

8 ounces warm, filtered water
1/3 cup fresh lemon juice
1 teaspoon Maca gelatinized powder
2 tablespoons apple cider vinegar (optional)
½-1 tablespoon MCT oil (optional)
Sweeten with stevia

1. Heat the water.
2. Squeeze the lemon into the water.
3. Mix together the lemon, apple cider vinegar, water, Maca powder, and MCT oil until well blended and no lumps appear.
4. Sweeten with stevia to taste.

Drink this concoction down while warm first thing in the morning to get the liver cleansing benefits of the lemon, smooth elimination from the MCT oil and apple cider vinegar, and the energy boost from the Maca powder. You can decide whether you wish to include the MCT oil or not but I like to use it for smooth elimination. (Sometimes I back it down to ½ tablespoon or add more water because I can taste the MCT oil.)

MCT (Medium Chain Triglycerides) oil is excellent for athletes to take because it provides quick energy since it bypasses digestion, goes straight to the liver, and is used just like glucose even though it is fat from coconut oil.

4
Intuition

Go Old School

The side of me that only wants the best for you must tell you the truth right now. I'm going to go rogue. Ditch your many gadgets and go old school. You can spend an exorbitant amount of time with a wide array of gadgets. I find that if you are constantly checking them, then you're wasting precious workout time. The biggest reason people give for missing a workout is lack of time. Now don't get me wrong. Gadgets are useful. They can measure heart rate, calories burned, and the effort you've put into your workout. When training, you may perceive your heart rate is higher than it is. When you have the accuracy of a heart rate monitor you may find you have to work a lot harder to get into the target zone. In addition, counting your steps may cause you to increase your activity level. So, yes, there are benefits to gadgets, but they're not the end-all be-all. I've had clients that were sitting on the couch not doing anything but grading papers and their device calculated that they took 2000 steps. The other problem is that many people think calories-in versus calories-out is an exact science. This method doesn't take into consideration what type of calories you're eating. There is a big difference between eating Oreos that are full of refined sugar and eating an apple. When you eat too much sugar it produces insulin which causes you to store fat. That is one of the biggest reasons you want to eat low glycemic foods and preferably with good fat and fiber to slow down the absorption of sugar into the bloodstream. The Sisterhood of S.W.E.A.T. focuses on what type of calories you're eating, when you're eating, what you're combining, and eating everything fresh and unprocessed. I don't want you eating anything from a box that lasts on the shelf for three years. Shop the outer aisles of the grocery store. If it swims in the sea, flies in the air or grows in the ground and it's organic, you can eat it. 85% of your results come from what you put in your mouth anyway! So go old school and take your pulse.

Go With Your Gut

The other thing that fit trackers don't take into account is that when you have bad gut bacteria you have to eat 30% less and work out 30% harder to get the same results as someone that has the correct amount of flora in their gut. The gut is responsible for a lot. It processes chemicals, digests food, initiates elimination, absorbs nutrients, and controls many of your emotions. 95% of your serotonin levels are located in your bowels. In the future, it may benefit you to pay attention to your gut feelings in more ways than one. There are so many studies out there now to prove how important it is to take a good probiotic. Your digestive health has a significant impact on weight loss. It is estimated that 80% of your immune system is located in your digestive system (Mercola). I think it is imperative to your overall health, immune system, and weight loss goals to take a good probiotic. If you don't have a good balance of intestinal flora in the gut then you're more likely to have weight gain. It is a telltale sign when you have a lot of weight gain around the middle that you're probably not digesting and eliminating your food properly. If you are eating too much sugar or have taken a lot of antibiotics, you may have an overgrowth of yeast or Candida in the body. If you suffer from an overgrowth of yeast it can cause numerous symptoms such as brain fog, bloating, and weight gain to name a few. Taking regular probiotics can help to restore gut health. At least 30% of neurotransmitters that send messages to the brain from your cells and hormone receptors come from your gastrointestinal lining which is why the gut is sometimes referred to as the "second brain." It may surprise you to know that feelings of happiness or misery come from your gut. Major neurotransmitters like serotonin, dopamine, glutamate, norepinephrine and nitric oxide are found in the gut. When gut health is out of balance this can greatly affect your weight loss, motivation, and drive.

Gut Health Supplements

The supplement, HCl, is something that your body naturally makes and can help with digestion. Once you hit the age of forty, the HCl in your body diminishes. Most arthritis sufferers are low in HCl. When you have low amounts of HCl, toxins may be stored more readily because they have nowhere to go. When you don't digest or eliminate properly, toxins can store in the joints. A lot of the time, people are diagnosed with acid reflux and think they need to take an antacid. In actuality, the problem may be that they don't have enough acid to digest their food, not that they have too much acid. Taking an antacid may cause chronic lower stomach acid which will only exasperate the problem. Dr. Mercola explains that, "Acid Reflux is a condition in which the acid in your stomach is coming out where it's supposed to remain. H-Pylori in your gut can cause inflammation and be one of the contributing factors to acid reflux as well as a Hiatal Hernia" (Mercola). Though HCl is a natural substance, it is an acid that helps with digestion and can help eliminate H-Pylori. I recommend taking it with your heavier meals. You will want to start with the recommend dosage on the bottle. A simple way to tell if you are taking too much is to monitor how your stomach feels. If you feel a warm or burning sensation, you know to back down on the dosage.

My favorite brand of probiotics is Dr. Ohhira's Probiotics Professional Formula capsules by Essential Formulas. What I like best about this brand is the product is made from whole foods, it is six times stronger than any known bacteria, you don't have to refrigerate it, it actually helps you produce your own natural flora, balances your hormones, helps digest your protein, enhances athletic performance, and gets rid of lactic acid. Another probiotic that I find very effective that is new on the market is REGACTIV. This particular probiotic strain makes its own antioxidants and supports healthy glutathione levels which are crucial for healthy liver function.

Trust Your Gut

You know that feeling when alarm bells go off and you just feel something in your gut, go with that. Don't second guess yourself. Gut feelings are pretty powerful. Our gut thinks for itself, the brain doesn't even have to send signals to the gut. The gut has a mind of its own. Listen to your gut instincts and tune in to them. Always trust your instincts; they will save you time and time again from a lot of grief and inconvenience. A lot of the time we don't trust our instincts because what they are telling us doesn't coincide with any facts that we have or we feel that we don't have enough information to go on. Another reason we find it so hard to trust our gut instincts is they don't always follow along a logical path of reason, they just are. I believe this can be attributed to the things we can't see such as our sixth sense, otherwise called your instincts or intuition.

Instincts

Sometimes your instincts are screaming so loud but you refuse to listen because it's embarrassing. I remember one time I had a date that was going to come and pick me up for the first time at my parents' house. Hours before the date I wanted to cancel or call and say I was going to drive myself. I just didn't have a good feeling about it. No explanation, just that gut feeling kicking in hard. I was just about to call him and say I would just meet him when he showed up at my door an hour and a half early. I felt stuck so I went. As the date progressed, he had all of his friends come up to me to tell me what a great guy he was. As an added bonus, every time he threw a dart, he tried to plant a kiss on me like I was his property. I got very uncomfortable and wanted to find an excuse to leave. I was always the nice, polite girl so I found it very hard to let someone down. I decided to fake a stomachache. As he was driving me home, I realized he wasn't taking me there. I started to get worried the farther we went in the wrong direction.

"Where are we going?" I asked.

49

"I have some apple cider at my house that I want to give to your kids," he said.

Possible excuse, right? My gut feelings were really kicking in hard at this point. I was beginning to get scared. Still, the nice girl in me wanted to give him the benefit of the doubt. Maybe he really did have apple cider he wanted to give my kids? I went in and then he had some something he wanted to show me, some kind of pictures in his photo album. Pretty soon the advances started, as you can well imagine. He told me he wanted to kidnap me and keep me and wanted to know if I would go up and help him make his bed?

"Um, I made my bed today all by myself. I'm pretty sure you can make yours," I said.

He asked me in a threatening sort of tone if I really wanted to go home. "Because you have a stomachache, right? It's not because you don't like me, is it?" he asked.

At this point, I really wanted out of there and I was scared. Yes, I absolutely have a stomachache. In fact, I think I'm going to puke. I got up and scrambled for the door as fast as I could. Thank God it was unlocked. I burst out of the door and did my best throwing up job ever. Finally, he agreed to take me home. Thank goodness I arrived at my door safely, no thanks to my own naivety. I was living with my parents after my divorce because there were still concerns for my safety at the time. I hadn't really dated much before my first marriage so I was wet behind the ears.

Mother's Intuition

I had come home from work early and I just had this unshakable feeling about my children so I asked my mother where they were.

> "Oh, they are at a neighbor's house down the street," she assured me.
> "What neighbor's house?" I asked.

I rushed right down to that neighbor's house because I did not know them, went in, and introduced myself. When I met the father, I took one look at him, looked into his eyes, and I knew I did not want my children in that house ever. I told my mother the children were only allowed to play together outside. My children were never to go in that house again under any circumstances.

Only a week later, the neighbor's wife shot him dead in that house. I am so glad that I trusted my instincts. Apparently he was an abuser and things got out of hand. I'm so glad my children weren't around when that unfolded.

These stories are great lessons on trusting your gut. Go with your intuition and internal instincts. Better to be embarrassed and alive then polite and dead.

Self-Health

Western medicine, generally speaking, only looks at the symptom of what's wrong and then gives the patient a medicine with side effects ten times worse than the problem. Now, with the affordable healthcare act (that wording alone is a joke), our healthcare is about to go through the roof.

So, I must ask this question: Have you ever considered taking charge of your own health? I, for one, do not want to leave my health in the hands of the Federal Government. I am fifty-three years old, not on medication of any kind, and I go to a holistic doctor which I pay for out of pocket. My holistic doctor always gives natural solutions. I truly believe an ounce of prevention is worth a pound of cure. I eat a whole foods diet, stay away from anything overly processed as much as possible, and I make sure to break a sweat daily.

Most chronic diseases can be prevented by just managing what goes in your mouth. Diabetes, heart disease, high blood pressure, obesity, and cigarette induced lung cancer, in many cases, are entirely preventable. I heard this statement recently and wholeheartedly agree: Food is the most abused anxiety drug and exercise the most underutilized antidepressant. The alternative is also true: Food can be your medicine and exercise your drug. It is worth taking the time to be mindful of what you eat. Healthy meals aren't just going to magically appear in front of you so you must be intentional in your choices. I ask people all the time where they live and they reply with an address, but the reality is that we live in our body and that is the home we better take care of.

The real truth about healthcare is that it starts with you. Be your own best friend. Make the choice today to take your power back and to begin investing your time into doing your own research on the benefits and healing properties of natural food. With a natural foods focus, better health and weight loss are just byproducts. Make yourself a priority. Any age rocks when you're healthy and you fuel your body with natural substances. Reach your goals and your dreams naturally by cutting all of the crap out of your diet and breaking a sweat daily.

Supplements

I'm not a big believer in taking an excessive amount of supplements but I do believe in those that enhance what you cannot get from food. I think if you've taken something for two to three weeks and you don't notice any good out of it, it's probably a wasted supplement. Too many supplements = expensive pee. The best thing you can do is to get a blood test and a tissue mineral analysis so you know exactly what you're lacking and what your body needs so that you're not guessing at it. The following is a list of some of the things that I don't like to go without.

*Consult with your doctor before the use of any supplement.

1. HCl - The supplement, HCl, is something that your body naturally makes and can help with digestion. Once you hit the age of forty, the HCl in your body diminishes. Most arthritis sufferers are low in HCl. When you have low amounts of HCl, toxins may be stored more readily because they have nowhere to go. When you don't digest or eliminate properly, toxins can store in the joints. A lot of the time, people are diagnosed with acid reflux and think they need to take an antacid. In actuality, the problem may be that they don't have enough acid to digest their food, not that they have too much acid. Taking an antacid may cause chronic lower stomach acid which will only exasperate the problem. Though HCl is a natural substance, it is an acid that helps with digestion and can help eliminate H-Pylori. I recommend taking it with your heavier meals. You will want to start with the recommend dosage on the bottle. A simple way to tell if you are taking too much is to monitor how your stomach feels. If you feel a warm or burning sensation, you know to back down on the dosage.

2. Probiotics - are live bacteria and yeasts that are good for your health, especially your digestive system. We usually think of bacteria as something that causes disease but your body is full of bacteria, both good and bad. Probiotics are often called "good" or "helpful" bacteria because they help keep your gut healthy.

3. BCAAs - improve exercise performance, endurance, and are helpful

for retaining muscle mass while dieting. BCAAs bypass the liver and gut, going directly into your bloodstream to be used as an immediate energy boost during your workouts.

4. Glutamine - is a natural food substance that fuels the brain, raises endorphin levels, and can help to balance moods by balancing blood sugar. Glutamine is also great for alleviating muscle soreness and sugar cravings.

5. Ashwagandha - is an adaptogen with healing benefits that are great for stress, fatigue, and energy. It stabilizes blood sugar, helps to lower cholesterol, and improves memory and concentration.

6. Maca - helps to decrease menopausal symptoms, depression, and balances hormones. It can also increase libido, energy levels, athletic performance, muscle building, and bone density. Though Maca helps energy levels, it does not place added stress on the adrenals and supports thyroid health.

7. Brewer's Yeast - has a high chromium content which helps to decrease blood sugar levels and is an excellent source of protein and B vitamins. Use in moderation.

5
Training Day

When, Where, Why, and How of Training

The little voice inside your head says, "It's early, dark, and cold outside." The temptation to pull the covers over your head and go back to bed when your alarm goes off for early morning exercise is very real. The little voice inside your head says, "It's raining. The instructor is probably going to cancel this morning anyway," or, "I'll get it in later today." Usually later never comes because something else gets in the way. In the early morning, there are fewer distractions.

One of the questions I'm asked a lot is whether it's better to work out in the morning, afternoon, or evening? Well, my first answer is: *Whenever you're willing to do it.* Doing some exercise is better than none at all. However, I am more of a morning advocate because the biggest problems I see are people making excuses, missing their workouts, and not being consistent. Things just get in the way. The statistics don't lie—90% of people that are consistent exercisers do it in the morning. Another plus for morning exercise is you're going to be more productive when starting your day. Getting up and getting your endorphins going naturally make you more energized.

When you have that little argument in your head, which voice wins? Every time you delay the start of your day and you say, "Awww..., just a few more minutes," you put your dreams on hold, the life you want to live, and the body you want to have.

Not all hours are created equal. Getting up before the rest of the world gives you a jump on your day. You get your day started off right. Early morning exercise amps up the metabolism and calorie burn for the rest of the day. Starting your day with a healthy mindset will make you more likely to eat right as well. Nothing and nobody is in your way in the early morning except you. So get out of your own way.

How Long and How Often Should I Work Out?

I am asked this question a lot. I'm from the school of thought that you should sweat and be active every day. One pitfall you definitely want to avoid is working out hard for one hour and then sitting all day long. It's what you do through the majority of the day that matters. I also don't encourage working out to the point of being so sore you can hardly move or do anything the next day. That's where you need to draw the line. It's what you do each day that matters. Consistency is king! How long you work out really depends on your goals. You can get a great workout in in a short amount of time if you stay focused and you work hard. I really think you can get a lot more done in the gym when you have a plan, you go in, and you kill it, rather than spending hours on end with no direction, just trying to burn calories. We eat far more often than we could ever train for so our time is better spent in the kitchen.

How Do I Know If I'm Overtraining?

The bottom line is you stop getting results. When it seems like you're going backwards and you dread every workout, you're overtraining and under resting. Overtraining is just as bad as undertraining, if not worse. When you over train, you begin breaking down the body and it becomes much easier to get injured. When you have a goal, it's easy to get overzealous and not know how much is enough. Your body works like a car engine—you've got to give it the right kind of fuel. Baby your body like you would a sports car. Treat it right and give it tune-ups and tender loving care.

Make Your Exercise Routine Excuse-Proof

1. I don't have time.

    Schedule your exercise time. Everyone has the same twenty-four hours in a day. Taking care of our health needs to be a priority that we don't skip. If we don't take care of ourselves, we won't be able to take care of anyone else. Americans, on a whole, spend an average of three to four hours a day watching TV or surfing the web. Surely we can find the time to take care of our health.

2. I have no energy.

    The more sedentary you are, the less energy you will have. The solution to a lack of energy is simple—just get up and get moving and soon you will become more energized. To gain energy, you must create it simply by moving more. Exercise doesn't need to be grueling. Make it doable and begin with just ten minutes of easy exercises. The more you do, the more you will be able to do.

3. I'm not seeing results.

    Sometimes it's hard when we are surrounded by the media's idea of what the perfect woman supposedly looks like. This often causes us to have unrealistic expectations and to become frustrated with ourselves when we are unable to achieve the same results. Many of the images we are faced with every day are computer generated, photoshopped, and downright deceptive. Don't define your results by trying to measure up to unrealistic media images. Try to measure your results by instead noticing the benefits that exercise provides such as more energy, fitting better into your clothes, weight loss, inch loss, sleeping better at night, mental alertness and clarity, fat loss, muscle gain, and feeling more fit.

4. I hate exercise.

    Find activities that you enjoy and then you will look forward to exercising and be much more likely to stick with it. When you do something you enjoy, it will feel less like exercise and much more like fun. Exercise shouldn't feel like drudgery but instead like an enjoyable interlude from your daily tasks.

5. The economy is so bad right now that I can't afford to spend time exercising.

Sitting around eating comfort food, watching endless hours of news, and constantly checking the stock reports isn't going to make things better. Instead, you will worry more about things that seem to be spiraling out of control. Be proactive and take charge of your health. Taking the time to exercise and to take care of yourself is totally in your hands. Exercising will relieve stress and anxiety and make you feel much more in control of things.

6. I am so out of shape that exercising just isn't going to make a difference.

It probably took you a while to get out of shape so it will take some time to get back into shape. Just take it one step at a time. Continually develop your base, begin with a ten minute exercise segment and then gradually increase your time three to five minutes each time you exercise. Keep doing ten minute sessions until you feel comfortable enough to increase to fifteen minute sessions, then twenty minutes, and before you know it, you will be able to work out for forty minutes without stopping.

6
Determination

Lose Fat Faster

Are you sweating? Is it hard to talk? Is it hard to breathe? Do you wonder when in the hell the torture is going to be over? If you answered, "Yes," then you're working hard enough to get results. Have proof that you're expending energy. Sweat is proof you've expended energy. Steady state cardio is just like it sounds, nice and steady. I recommend H.I.I.T./Functional Training two to three times a week. H.I.I.T. (High Intensity Interval Training) makes sure your body never gets used to a workout, your body cannot adapt, so you will always burn the maximum amount of calories. Therefore H.I.I.T./Functional Training is going to yield the greatest results long term.

Steady state has its place because you can't go 100 miles an hour all the time. Your central nervous system can only handle so much. That's why when you go hard in the gym for four days and then try to include two to three H.I.I.T. sessions, you struggle. When you overdo it, your body just wants to shut down. You know what I'm talking about—those workouts that you just hardly get through. You must work hard and then work easy and incorporate recovery time. The other beautiful thing about H.I.I.T. is that your sprint and my sprint aren't going to be the same. You may perceive running fifty yards at fifty seconds as fast while I may perceive ten seconds as fast. We both are right. We could both be expending the same calorie burn because we are both working at our maximum level. If you don't have much time, H.I.I.T. is perfect. Plus, with H.I.I.T. training, you can get a great workout in a short amount of time. Be careful not to overdo this style of training because it affects your central nervous system and may cause your cortisol levels to increase. Cortisol is an adrenal hormone which is released in response to fear or stress. It is activated by the flight or fight response. Increased cortisol levels from added stress of any kind can cause you to store fat around the middle or just in general all over the body. Over training essentially defeats the purpose of trying to lose fat stores. Remember, less is more when you start to think about increasing your training. Focusing on your diet to get lean will produce much better results than overtraining. The secret to a great physique is keeping a balance of progressive overload with periods of rest. You never want to place such a great amount of stress on your muscles that you cannot efficiently repair and recover.

Recommended Weekly Training SOS (Sisterhood of S.W.E.A.T.)

Functional training exercises mimic the way you move in everyday life to complete various tasks. Functional training is highly effective as opposed to exercises, such as a bicep curl, because we concentrate on whole body movements that fire more than one muscle group at a time, thus having a more metabolic effect.

1. 2-3 intense SOS H.I.I.T. cardio sessions a week, 30 min each.
2. 1-2 SOS functional training sessions, 60 min each.
3. 3-4 weight training sessions, 45-60 min each.

Benefits of H.I.I.T.:

1. Increase muscle mass
2. Lose fat faster
3. Increase the growth hormone
4. Boost metabolism
5. Torch a huge amount of calories in a small amount of time
6. Improve cardiovascular health
7. Boredom busting
8. Plateau busting

It's okay to be uncomfortable.

This came straight out of the mouth of one of my clients during a 6:00 am boot camp.

"I always believed in these articles that said something like, 'Do these ten things and you will be in shape,' or, 'Try these five moves to get great glutes.' There are no ten simple things that are going to get you in shape.

The one thing that I learned in the last two weeks is that little things don't work, and that if you want to achieve something, you have to jump in with both feet. The other thing I've learned is it's okay to be uncomfortable. I was all about feeling comfortable all the time and now I've found out that you just have to push through. You will be uncomfortable and it's okay."

She learned three very important things:

1. To be comfortable in your skin, you have to be willing to be uncomfortable during your workouts.

2. Do the work and you will achieve results.

3. Jump in with both feet and go after it.

Do the Work

To be a S.W.E.A.T. sister in the sisterhood, you've got to put in the sweat equity. Do the work! To get the body you want, you have to push harder than you ever have. You may say to yourself, "I've just not got it in me today," or, "I'm so tired." When it's workout day, you may not feel like doing it. You may be sluggish and sore as hell. You have to look at your end goal and push through it. We never regret the workouts we do. The workouts we regret are the ones we didn't do, the ones where we slacked off and gave ourselves a pass not to push hard or do as many reps because we didn't feel like it. When you don't feel like working out, you have to push through, so that at the end of the day, you can achieve your goals. It's about having a plan and following it. Get away from the mentality of, "Well, I only have thirty minutes so no sense in exercising and wasting my time." Lose the excuse you tell yourself when you say, "I'm going on vacation in a week so I don't see what I can get done in a week. I'll just wait until I get back." Get up, get moving, and do the work. Build up some sweat equity. It's what you do every day and how active you are on the whole that adds up. Move every day and do something that makes you sweat. Something is always worth it. The workouts you do, the workouts you don't do, they all add up in the long run.

Use your common sense and good judgment when working out.

Don't work out if you have the following:

1. The flu

2. A fever

3. Injuries

4. Doctor's advice to not exercise

5. A cold

Hit It until You Quit It

Seriously, have you ever been to a gym where you see people just barely moving on the treadmill, reading a book, doing a set then talking, or just wandering around like they're lost? Then they wonder why they have been spending so much time at the gym but they're not getting any results. We only have so much time in the day to get our workouts done so they need to be spot on. No lollygagging around when you go to the gym. Hit it until you quit it. By the time you have complained, dreaded it, and thought about it, you could've done it. Don't waste time.

1. Have a plan.

2. Wear headphones.

3. Work with intensity.

We have two types of muscle fibers: fast twitch (type 2) and slow twitch (type 1). It's important to get both of them to fire and engage 100%. Slow twitch muscles help enable long endurance feats such as distance running. Fast twitch muscles fatigue faster but are used in powerful bursts of movements like sprinting. Fast twitch muscles are the largest and most powerful in the body, but as we age, they are also the most neglected. In the Sisterhood of S.W.E.A.T. Exercise Selection, we are almost always going to work some fast twitch muscle. To have the body of an athlete, you must train like an athlete. During athletic movements, there are bursts of speed as well as feats of endurance where you engage all of your muscle groups and they fire more as a whole. Fast twitch fiber stores a lot of carbohydrates, carries less fat, and is more metabolic. The lack of fast twitch muscle fiber is why we begin to notice that we aren't as "tight" as we used to be.

Fire Up - Fast Twitch

1. Go Heavy (Lift heavier weights, but not at the sacrifice of good form.)
2. Do Plyometrics
3. Run Sprints
4. H.I.I.T.
5. Bootcamp

Fire Up - Slow Twitch

1. Jogging
2. Elliptical
3. Cycling
4. Walking
5. Weight Training (light weight, high reps)

Slow twitch muscle is great for endurance and burning fat but not as effective as fast twitch fibers for the building of long lean muscle. That is why you need both and we will incorporate this theory in our training.

To increase your metabolism and aid in recovery, try adding a few short, low intensity sessions to your training each week. Train hard, then easy. The low intensity training sessions will recruit your slow twitch muscle.

Doing full body workouts, such as our SOS functional training, will fire up more muscle groups at a time, ultimately burning more calories per workout session. When you decrease the total volume per muscle group, you will automatically increase the recovery rate.

Work around it!

If I had a nickel for every time I've heard, "But I can't do it because this aches and that aches," I would be rich. Work around it! There are plenty of things you can do. Stop focusing on what you can't do or soon you will be doing nothing. Feast your eyes on the end result or else all you will see is obstacles.

*Do not ignore chronic injuries, seek medical attention.

Kill the Cardio Beast Within

Seriously, I see people work out in the gym, logging in hours of time on all the cardio equipment, but spending very little time on resistance training and then wondering why their bodies never change.

Resistance/weight training is the key to changing your body. Although doing steady state cardio burns calories and makes you feel like you're losing weight, resistance/weight training is the key to changing and reshaping your body. The more muscle you have, the more calories you burn at rest. One pound of fat burns 5-10 calories at rest, but one pound of muscle burns 50-100 calories at rest. Which would you rather have? Muscle boosts your metabolism all day long, while cardio boosts it for just a few hours. I know that sometimes women get scared when I mention the word muscle. They start to envision themselves all big, thick, and bulging. Not to worry—only 4% of women develop large muscles. The majority of us simply don't have enough testosterone for that phenomenon to occur. Compared by volume, muscle weighs more than fat. This is why a person with higher body fat will float more easily than a person with more muscle. Muscle is much more condensed and it takes up a lot less space than fat. So when you are dropping fat and adding muscle, you may not notice a difference on the scale even though you notice a change in your clothes and you look leaner in the mirror. Too many people focus on losing weight when they should really concentrate on gaining muscle. Adding muscle is the quickest and most effective way to turn your body into a fat burning machine. Lean muscle is metabolically active and burns calories even when you're vegging out or catching some Zzz's. Sure, doing steady state or slow motion cardio burns calories, but which is more important—what your body burns in an hour or what it burns all day long?

The bottom line is that you will be burning calories all day long at a more rapid rate if you harbor a lot of lean muscle mass. Long slow distance cardio (LSD) may also accelerate the aging process as it causes inflammation and too much oxidative stress on your body. Less is definitely more in the scheme of things. Too much cardio and overtraining will actually decrease power and speed. A study from 1976 in the Journal of Applied Psychology found that you secrete two times the cortisol levels at thirty minutes of exercise compared to ten minutes (Sheridan). Too much cortisol promotes fat storage and will tear down your muscle. All that being said, we will do some steady state cardio because it has its place. Variety is the name of the game. Alternating steady state cardio with H.I.I.T training will prevent you from inflicting as much wear and tear on the body as well as keep workouts interesting. It is good to have an interactive balance in your exercise regimen as our bodies are highly adaptable to whatever we do. The trick is to mix it up so you get the best results and look forward to your individual exercise time.

7
No Easy Way Out

No Magic Pill

I hate it when the mainstream media recommends this product and that quick-fix or miracle solution for what ails you. My clients come to me and want to know if it will be the solution to their problems. A magic pill is not going negate eating an entire box of doughnuts. The truth is, it's really basic. Sweat every day, eat non-processed foods, drink clean water, sleep, and rid yourself of toxins and stress.

What most people don't realize when trying to achieve weight loss is that eating right, not exercise, is responsible for 75% of their results. More often than not people will over exercise and under eat to get the weight off. That might work at first but will fail long-term. Health and fitness are a total package.

Don't fall for gimmicks, quick fixes, product claims, and marketing schemes. My experience with fat burners and/or stimulants hasn't been a good one. I started using them many years ago when a gym owner suggested they would help me burn fat. I was new at the fitness game and I figured he would know what he was talking about since he was buff and owned a gym, right? Too often, people seek others for advice without knowing what their true qualifications are.

Fat Burners

Fat burners took more from me than they ever gave. This was when ephedrine was all the rage. Now you can't even put ephedrine on the shelf because people use it to make meth. The over-the-counter stimulants and the ephedrine became such a crutch for me that I couldn't start my day without them because I was addicted to them. It was in the same way many people are addicted to caffeine and sugar. I thought it was giving me energy to get through a very physical day and to do all the activities I had on my plate as an overachiever. Equally, I thought that taking fat burners were helping me to keep fat off, stay lean, and lose weight. To put it mildly, my adrenals got so burnt out from the overstimulation of the "magic pill" (that was supposedly safe), I don't know how they ever fired up again. The catch 22 with fat burners is that you may start off burning fat in the beginning and it's great, but soon you're going to get addicted and feel that you need them. You will be addicted to the quick fix, the energy, and the feeling that they're helping you. Because you think they work, you'll continue to take them and maybe even up your dose when you notice they're not doing as much for you as they did in the beginning. Before you know it, you've set yourself up for adrenal burnout. When your adrenals slow down, your metabolism comes to an absolute standstill. Fat burners are such jokes. I am so much smaller, healthier, and have endless energy since I got off the fat burners and got onto the nutrition train. Looking great on the outside means nothing if you damage your health. You can't put that genie back in the bottle.

Contrary to many dieting ads, there are no shortcuts or magic pills on the road to ultimate health. Longevity doesn't come in a pill bottle. If it did, we would all be taking it. A lifestyle change is what it takes to be in charge of your own future health's destination. Wouldn't it be great if we could decide how quickly we aged? Well, according to multitudes of research on aging, we can. The decision is really in our hands. We just have to take a few simple steps to begin our quest.

Food Choices Matter

When you're going to take a bite of something, you may say to yourself, "A little bit of this and that doesn't matter." A little bit does matter and if tracked, can add up to an extra 10-15 pounds of weight gain each year. Did you know that according to the Calorie Control Council that the average holiday meal such as Thanksgiving dinner contains 4,500 calories and 229 grams of fat? This is the average amount Americans consume at a typical Thanksgiving dinner. People come to me because they have heart disease, they've had a stroke, high cholesterol, and clogged arteries. "An ounce of prevention is worth a pound of cure." These diseases are, for the most part, entirely preventable. So yes, your food choices do matter. Don't kid yourself. It's what you do the majority of the time that matters.

If you eat cheat meals every weekend and wonder why you may not be losing weight—there are 365 days in a year, 104 of them are on the weekend which is roughly a third of the year. With 261 days dedicated to fitness and 104 dedicated to indulging, your results will drastically suffer.

Did you know that eating an extra 100 calories a day will add ten pounds in one year?! Choose your indulgences wisely. Weekends make up over 104 days a year—a heck of a lot of cheat meals could go down in that time frame. You can have a treat but I wouldn't say have a season of treats. My suggestion is to try reducing it to one cheat meal versus the whole weekend so that you don't sabotage your fitness goals. For the purpose of this book, we will incorporate Sunday Funday. You will be able to eat foods on Sunday in any order you choose from the grocery list and have one treat meal of your choice.

Why Journal?

I always have my health coaching clients fill out a daily food journal with workouts. I can directly correlate their results by how closely they follow their plan. When I receive regular journals and photo check-ins from my clients, I know that beyond a shadow of a doubt they will be soon sending me notes on how they've dropped a pant size or have shed weight. It is a game changer to have some sort of accountability. When you write down what you're eating, it is so much easier to track, see where you went wrong, and to make a change. It is proven that when you journal you will be 50% more likely to succeed. Up your success rate and write it down!

When you write things down, you will notice various behaviors that might be setting you back. Journaling allows for honesty with yourself. When you write down what you're doing, you can't lie to yourself as easily about why you're not getting results. For instance, you might be eating mindlessly while you watch TV and perhaps you're eating an entire bag of chips in a sitting. You may not notice that you ate an entire bag of chips every day for a month if you're not writing it down. What you do on a regular basis adds up, good or bad. Writing your goals down and keeping track of what you do is a simple process that yields significant rewards.

Why Journal?

1. Goal setting.
2. Accountability.
3. A measurement of where you started and where you are now.
4. Great for keeping track of where you are so you know where you could be going wrong with your exercise or diet plan.
5. An overall assessment and monitoring of your progress.
6. Honesty with yourself, enabling you to rein yourself in if you need to.
7. A reference point for why you may be succeeding or failing.

"Always carry a notebook. And I mean always. The short-term memory only retains information for three minutes; unless it is committed to paper, you can lose an idea for ever." ~Will Self

8
Cleanse and Detox

Cleanse Benefits - Year Round Cleanse

*Be sure to consult your doctor before beginning any new cleansing or fasting regimen. Cleanses are not intended for use by minors, pregnant or nursing women, individuals with any type of health/medical condition or users of prescription drugs. Such individuals are strongly advised to seek professional (medical) advice prior to initiating any form of cleansing, fasting, weight loss effort or regimen. Fasting is to be discouraged before or after surgery as it might interfere with the body's healing process.

*You should not participate in the detox if you have been diagnosed with any type of disease or immune disorder.

~Do not take supplements during this time other than Dr. Ohhira's probiotics.

Welcome to the seven day, year round cleanse - Cleanse Benefits

I originally constructed Cleanse Benefits to take place right after the New Year when I had a feeling we could all do with a little cleanse/detox. When I realized how toxic our world had become, I recognized that we could all use a cleanse periodically throughout the year. So I created Cleanse Benefits, the seven day, all year round cleanse.

Detoxification is a process to cleanse the body of impurities and the toxic load accumulated from living in an environment that is laden with chemically processed foods, pesticides, fake food substances, and preservatives. During complete detox days, you will want to rest in order to enable the body's organs to release toxins and cleanse more effectively. Your body will be working hard to rid itself of all chemical buildup and in order for this to happen, detoxifying needs to be your main focus. You don't want your body to be busy doing too many things during this time. The detoxification process is hard enough on the body without adding intense workouts to the mix. You are going to give your body and digestive system a long needed rest and a good house cleaning. Before starting the actual detox process, you will ease into it by eliminating anything overly processed. It is important to start with at least one week on The Basic Plan to clean up your diet before beginning the Cleanse Benefits program. Equally important will be keeping your diet clean once the cleanse is completed.

During the detox you will take the pressure off of your digestive load by avoiding all meat, poultry, fish, eggs, and dairy products, as well as fried foods and nuts. Next, you will reduce the intake of toxic substances by eliminating alcohol, tobacco, sweets, and junk food, all of which act as toxins in the body and are obstacles to the cleansing process. During the detox you will consume a diet high in fresh fruit and vegetables that are loaded with vitamins, minerals, phytochemicals and antioxidants. You are giving the digestive system a rest in order to enable the potent cleansing ingredients to take effect. The seven day time frame is necessary because it is takes a while to clean the blood and body of toxins and impurities. It is equally important to de-stress during the detox by including lighter activities such as yoga and walking and limit intense exercise so your system can effectively detox.

11 Signs You May Need to Detox:

- Bloating
- Weight gain
- Muffin top
- Cellulite
- Brain fog
- Memory loss
- Fatigue
- PMS
- Menopausal symptoms
- Mood swings
- Indigestion

Easy Pre-Cleanse

For the pre-cleanse, there are two options. Choose your preference, both options work. My advice is to choose the option you will do and can stick with because a plan only works if you are "werking it, girl."

Option 1- You may follow one week of The Basic Plan on page 130 as a pre-cleanse.

Option 2- (For women on-the-go) I prefer that you get your nutrition directly from food but I know what type of universe we live in and the cleanest shakes for convenience sake are Isagenix. For women on-the-go, this is just a very simple pre-cleanse.

Women On-the-Go 1 Week Pre-Cleanse

The Basic Plan Chart is listed on page 128. Each letter stands for a food group. The Women On-the-Go Pre-Cleanse serving amounts are listed below and they are different amounts than the ones listed on The Basic Plan S.W.E.A.T chart. Women on-the-go will also only have four meals instead of six. This is perfect for those of you that struggle to get all of your meals in. To order your Isagenix products for the Women On-the-Go Pre-Cleanse, go to http://lindalu7.isagenix.com/

P-Proteins, V-Vegetables, F-Fruits, C-Carbs, GF-Good Fats

1. **P. V. F. C. GF.** = 1 Isa-lean Pro Meal Replacement Shake = approximately 280 calories

2. **P. C. V.** = 1 low glycemic lean meal, 400-600 Calories
   P - 6 ounce protein, C - ¼ cup carb, V - 2 cups vegetables

   Example: **P** - One 6 ounce organic chicken breast, **A** - ¼ cup quinoa, **W** - 2 cups green beans = approximately 600 calories

3. **P. V. F. C. GF.** = 1 Isa-lean Pro Meal Replacement Shake = approximately 280 calories

4. **P. C. V.** = 1 low glycemic lean meal, 400-600 Calories
   P - 6 ounce protein, C - ¼ cup carb, V - 2 cups vegetables

   Example: **P** - One 6 ounce organic bison burger, **C** - ¼ cup sweet potato, **V** - 2 cups broccoli = approximately 600 calories

Cleanse Benefits-

1. Boosts energy
2. Rids the body of toxins and waste
3. Helps with weight loss
4. Strengthens the body's immune system
5. Clears the skin

6. Clears mental fogginess
7. Aids in digestion
8. Promotes healing
9. Diminishes the appearance of cellulite
10. Balances hormones
11. Helps reduce hot flashes
12. Helps to reduce arthritis pain
13. Fights inflammation

The 7 Day Cleanse Benefits in a Nutshell

Pre-Cleanse

It is important to start with at least one to two weeks on The Basic Plan or Women On-the-Go to clean up your diet before beginning the Cleanse Benefits Program. It is equally important to keep your diet clean once the cleanse is completed. Don't just jump back into mainstream eating or a lot of unhealthy food choices because it could make you end up feeling sick. Besides, going straight back to old habits defeats the entire purpose of cleansing.

Days 1-4: Complete Detox

Day 5: Smoothies

Days 6 & 7: Cleansing Soup Recipe

Detox - Complete Detox Days 1-4

1. Drink Smooth Moves Tea. The night before you begin your cleanse, drink 1 cup of Smooth Moves Tea. The Smooth Moves comes in a variety of flavors, pick your favorite. Steep for 10-15 minutes.

2. Drink 6-10 servings of the Cleanse Benefits Cocktail (recipe to follow) throughout the day. You can purchase the Convenient Organic Lemonade Vibrant Diet Cleanse by Vibrant Health in a convenient

canister at Whole Foods or online at http://www.vibranthealth.us

3. Drink water or the Cleanse Water as needed.

4. The Cleanse Water and Cleanse Benefits Cocktail work as a prebiotic followed by your choice of probiotic supplement (such as Dr. Ohhira's probiotics).

5. Finish the day with a cup of herbal tea or laxative tea before bedtime.

6. Organic Coffee is allowed in moderation.

Repeat this for 1-4 days. On the last night, it is not necessary to drink the laxative tea. The Cleanse Benefits Cocktail will have a little zing to it. You may dilute it with more water if desired. It will grow on you. The cayenne pepper decreases appetite and revs up the metabolism. The smoothies section may be started early if you get too hungry to continue the whole 1-4 days. Even one day of a complete cleanse is beneficial. Listen to your body.

Detox - Day 5

On the first day after the complete detox days are finished,

1. Drink smoothies (recipes below).

2. Alternate Smoothies with fresh squeezed orange juice throughout the day.

3. Take your choice of probiotic.

4. Drink one cup of ginger, chamomile, or peppermint tea (great for bloating, irritable bowel, digestion, calming, and removing toxic waste from the body). Steep for 10-15 minutes.

5. Drink the Cleanse Water throughout the day.

Detox - Day 6

On the second day after the complete detox days are finished,
(You can eat as much of the Cleansing Soup as you want depending on how hungry you are. Take it slow as it is essentially the first solid food you will have had in a while.)

1. Drink fresh squeezed orange juice in the morning.

2. For lunch, have the Cleansing Soup (recipe below).

3. For dinner, have the Cleansing Soup. Rye wafers can be eaten with the soup, but sparingly.

4. Take your choice of Probiotic.

5. Drink the Cleanse Water throughout the day.

6. Drink one cup of ginger, chamomile, or peppermint tea (great for bloating, irritable bowel, digestion, calming, and removing toxic waste from the body). Steep for 10-15 minutes.

Detox-Day 7

(You can eat as much the Cleansing Soup as you want, again depending on how hungry you are.)

1. Fresh squeezed orange juice in the morning.

2. The Cleansing Soup for lunch.

3. Load up with raw fruits and veggies for dinner.

4. Take your choice of probiotic. Normal eating will be resumed the next day.

5. Drink the Cleanse Water throughout the day.

6. Drink one cup of ginger, chamomile, or peppermint tea (great for bloating, irritable bowel, digestion, calming, and removing toxic waste from the body). Steep for 10-15 minutes.

When you come off of the cleanse and begin putting food back into your system after depriving it of solid substances for three days, you could feel nauseated. You will definitely feel fuller with much smaller portion sizes so go easy at first. This goes with any fast (depriving your body of solid food for any period of time)! Part of this cleanse is to start tuning into your body and what it's telling you, so LISTEN! Everyone's experience will be different, so do what you feel is right for you.

Listen to your body! It is not necessary to drink the laxative tea—the Cleanse Benefits Cocktail by itself will work as a cleansing agent. Herbal tea and the Cleanse Water used in conjunction with the Cleanse Benefits Cocktail on a daily basis speeds up the cleansing process. The laxative tea may cause stomach cramps which is okay. If the cramps become unbearable, then try skipping the tea one night. If it continues to cause pain, then skip it all together. The tea is just to help get things moving. *If diarrhea occurs after taking the tea, stop taking the tea until the diarrhea dissipates.*

Cleanse Benefits

Cleanse, alkalize, rejuvenate and receive some of the benefits listed below. Any time of year is a great time to cleanse and to adapt to new, healthier habits. You will consume juices, hot teas, hot soups and many ingredients that will help flush out your system of toxins.

The healthy Cleanse Benefits Cocktail will have similar benefits to the staple beverage of Stanley Burroughs' Master Cleanse with lemon juice, cayenne pepper, and maple syrup!

Lemon juice - The lemon will help to cleanse the liver and has an alkalizing effect even though it's acidic. In the body, lemon turns to alkaline ash. The liver, which is the main detoxifying organ in the body, has so many functions, three of which are to filter your blood, store glycogen, and create a digestive substance called bile. If the liver is overloaded with toxins, it can't break down fat. The lemon juice will stimulate the liver to create bile which helps to break down fat.

Cinnamon, cloves, and maple syrup - These help to keep your blood sugar from dropping and are loaded with minerals. Cinnamon can also help to alleviate the pain caused by arthritis. A study out of Kansas University found that one teaspoon of cinnamon added to juice killed 99.5% of bacteria in the juice within three days (Reuters). Cloves are known to have antiviral and antifungal properties.

Ginger - Ginger is a powerful anti-inflammatory herb that also aids in digestion. Ginger is also great for arthritis sufferers.

Cayenne pepper - Cayenne adds heat, increases thermogenesis (which boosts your metabolism), aids in breaking down mucus buildup, and starts the cleansing process.

Unsweetened apple juice - Apple juice is a cleanser as well as a natural sweetener.

Blueberry, cranberry and pomegranate juice – All three juices are loaded with both vitamins A and C and a multitude of antioxidants that will act as natural diuretics, flushing out all excess water. The vitamin C in these juices can increase the body's ability to emulsify fat by as much as 30%.

Lemon juice, blueberry juice, and cayenne pepper – The three ingredients also help to break down fat. They help with digestion and help you to lose weight. If your digestive system is stagnant then it'll be next to impossible to lose weight—that is why we're incorporating the lemon juice and the apple cider vinegar as well as the cayenne pepper.

Blueberries, strawberries, and raspberries - These fruits are extremely low in calories (one half cup has approximately 40 calories). Blueberries protect against short-term memory loss and lower cholesterol. Berries are also known as blood purifiers. They contain many antioxidants that are known to help protect your body from heart disease and cancer. Berries also keep bacteria from sticking to the wall of the bladder so they work to prevent urinary tract infections. They can also reduce high blood pressure, combat fatigue, prevent colds, and reduce bad breath.

Oranges - Oranges are loaded with fiber, vitamin C, and powerful antioxidants. Eating oranges also helps to relieve constipation and lower cholesterol.

Grapefruit - Researchers at the famous Scripps Clinic in La Jolla, California found that eating half a grapefruit three times a day resulted in 800% more weight loss than those who skipped it completely (Gittleman). (Note: grapefruit may alter the effect of certain prescription medicines. Please consult your physician before consuming grapefruit or grapefruit juice.)

Spinach and kale - Both are loaded with vitamins and minerals and pack a powerful punch in the antioxidant department. While kale is loaded with vitamins A, K, and C, iron, bioavailable calcium, and has higher protein, spinach has 15% of your RDA in iron and is packed with magnesium and fiber. Spinach also has protein and a substance called oxalate which may keep you from absorbing some of it's natural calcium.

Carrot juice - Carrot juice provides a significant amount of A, B, and K vitamins, macronutrients, and minerals. Fresh carrot juice is a sweet tasting treat.

Daikon radish - According to traditional Chinese medicine, daikon radish is a fat flusher and fat metabolizer. Daikon is also known to aid in digestion, relieve fatigue, and for their ability to cleanse the blood and body.

Frequently Asked Questions and Concerns:

"Can I eat anything during the detox?"

The goal of the detox is to eliminate anything that the body has to work to digest in order to cleanse your entire system of impurities. If you still feel that you need to eat something, try adding the Cleansing Soup or a smoothie.

"I don't know if I can do this!"

A cleanse is a mind-body experience. It is essential that you give yourself lots of rest and relaxation during this time. It really isn't too bad. The Cleanse Benefits Cocktail keeps you from having cravings or being hungry.

"What if I want hot food?"

This is usually a reason for sabotaging the detox, especially during cold weather. You can try heating the Cleanse Benefits Cocktail, have some vegetable broth, or the Cleansing Soup to keep yourself warm and mineralized during the detox.

"How many fruit smoothies can I have on smoothie day?"

As many as you want. The smoothies are low calorie and will mainly have a flushing effect through your system since they are made entirely from fresh fruit.

"How many servings of the Cleansing Soup can I have?"

As many servings as you want. The soup is low calorie and very filling. It will just have a cleansing effect through your system as it is made mostly of broth and vegetables.

"How much orange juice can I have a day?"

Limit your orange juice to two cups (or 16 ounces) a day.

"Can I still drink the Cleanse Water when I'm finished with the cleanse? How much can I have?"

Yes. 64 ounces a day.

"How often should I cleanse?"

Four times a year, with the seasons.

Detox Recipes

Cleanse Juice, Day 1-4

Cleanse Benefits Cocktail

Prep time: 5 minutes
Cook time: 25 minutes

Step 1: Follow the instructions below to create the juice for the Cleanse Benefits Cocktail. Makes 2 quarts.

Step 2: When you are ready to enjoy a cocktail, mix 1 scoop of the Convenient Organic Lemonade Vibrant Diet Cleanse by Vibrant Health into each 8 ounce glass of juice. You can order online or find it at Whole Foods.

Ingredients:

1 cup of Knudsen's blueberry juice

1 cup of Knudsen's unsweetened pomegranate juice

8 cups of purified water

¾ cup of 100% fresh orange juice

½ cup apple juice

1 teaspoon cinnamon

1 teaspoon ginger

¼ teaspoon cloves

12 drops liquid stevia, or to taste

Instructions:
1. In a large pot, combine blueberry, pomegranate, apple and orange juice.
2. Bring to a boil.
3. Reduce the heat to a simmer and add cinnamon, ginger and cloves.
4. Simmer for 5 minutes, stirring occasionally.
Serve warm or cold.

Cleanse Water

1 cup Knudsen's unsweetened blueberry juice or cook your own 1 cup fresh organic blueberries (until syrup like)

½ cup Santa Cruz lemon juice

1/8 teaspoon cayenne pepper

2 quarts water

Liquid stevia, sweeten to taste

Smoothies Section, Day 5

Berry Banana Smoothie

Makes 2 servings

Ingredients:

2 cups frozen organic blueberries

½ cup unsweetened cranberry juice

1 cup baby kale

1 banana, peeled

Instructions:
1.   Combine all ingredients in a blender and process until smooth.

Strawberry Grapefruit Smoothie

Makes 3 servings

Ingredients:

1 ruby red grapefruit, peeled and seeded

2 cups fresh or frozen strawberries

1 sweet apple, cored and chopped

1 teaspoon fresh ginger, in the tube

1 cup water

1 tablespoon Chia seed

Instructions:
1.   Combine all ingredients in a blender and process until smooth.

Strawberry Banana Smoothie

Makes 2 servings

1 teaspoon cacao powder

1 cup strawberries

1 banana

1 cup unsweetened coconut milk

½ tablespoon coconut oil, melted

Instructions:
1.   Combine all ingredients in a blender and process until smooth.

Berry-Orange Smoothie

Makes 2 servings

Ingredients:

2 navel oranges, peeled with seeds removed, cut into wedges

1 cup frozen blueberries

1 cup frozen raspberries

Instructions:
1.   Combine all ingredients in a blender and blend until smooth.

Berry-Green Smoothie

Makes 3 servings

1 cup berries

1 cup unsweetened coconut milk

1 cup baby spinach, washed

¼ cup unsweetened carrot juice

1 tablespoon ground flaxseeds

1 tablespoon lemon juice

1/2 cup ice cubes

Instructions:
1. Combine all ingredients in a blender and blend until smooth.

Cleansing Soup Recipe, Day 6 & 7

<u>Cleansing Soup</u>

Ingredients:

1 bag of organic carrots

1 onion

5 celery stalks

1 daikon radish, chopped

2 parsnips

1 bunch of kale, stems removed

½ head of cabbage, chopped

1 tablespoon parsley

1 teaspoon basil

1/2 cup uncooked brown rice

2 teaspoon garlic salt

1 teaspoon oregano

64 ounces organic chicken broth (no cane sugar added)

Instructions:
1. Chop all ingredients into bite size pieces.
2. Put all vegetables, rice, and seasonings into a large pot. Add chicken broth. Add additional water until all the vegetables are covered.
3. Bring to a boil. Cover and simmer on low for approximately 1 hour.

9
Eating for Health

Eat Carrots, Not Crap

I don't believe eating carrots will prohibit your weight loss progress. I know a lot of diets are very restrictive in that regard. People worry about eating a carrot or having a banana but then they stick an entire chocolate bar in their mouth. That's the same principle behind stepping over dollars to pick up pennies. When it comes to eating, sometimes you can just use your common sense. It's not a rigid set of rules and guidelines. It's what you do most of the time that sets you apart and helps you to get the results you're seeking. Yep, I'm pretty sure it's that banana you had that kept you from fitting into your pants. Not. I'm certain if it wasn't a banana, it must be all that fruit you ate. Not. You get the general idea. Stick to eating what swims in the sea, flies in the air, or grows in the ground and you'll be on the safe side (organic and non-GMO, of course). I am going to give you a general guideline of healthy eating, a base, so to speak. You want to have a healthy foundation, a method of eating. Eating healthy is not completely black and white. Sometimes you're going to want an apple or an extra piece of bread. You don't want to go completely stir crazy. You're going to have to allow yourself to have things when you need them. So eat carrots, not crap, when the occasion arises.

Get Out of the Drive-Thru
and Into the Kitchen

I hate to break it to you but if you want to lose weight, get in shape, or just live a healthy lifestyle, you're going to have to wrap your mind around the fact that you need to learn to prepare your food. It's not that hard. I know some of you are like, "I can't cook. I don't have time. It's too much trouble. Can I just stop at the drive-thru? What can I eat at the doughnut shop?" No. No. No. All no. It really takes much more time to get in your car, drive somewhere, wait in the line, and drive home, than it takes to prep your food. Live your life on purpose, be intentional about what you put in your mouth, and you'll get the results you intend.

The only person that is going to prepare your food the way that you want it is you. You're going to make sure that it's fresh, clean, cooked the way you like it, with all of the vitamins, nutrients, and minerals that you need. You're going to have a lot more control over your future health knowing what's in your food, for the most part. I'm pretty sure you're not going to inject it with extra fat, GMOs, sugar, or an overdose of salt, like you might get at a restaurant. It's pretty shocking to do a calorie count when you eat out. You will discover that entrees you would expect to be low calorie such as a shrimp dish with butter sauce, could end up being 900 calories. In addition, these dishes may include your full fat and sodium content for the entire day in one serving. I'm not big into calorie counting but it does matter. You definitely don't want to eat 1500 calories at one sitting. I want you to focus on volume and nutrients in your food such as three cups of broccoli with a little seasoning—perhaps a little salt and some good fat—not three cups of broccoli with sugar and a cup of butter. Eat volume, not calories. When you eat fibrous carbs, they will fill you up and be slow to absorb because of the fiber, thus leaving you full longer. There is a notable difference in eating broccoli versus a chocolate chip cookie. Highly processed foods are stripped of everything good and will leave you wanting more. White bread is twice dead. I'm not saying you can never eat out at a restaurant, because you can, and I will teach you how to do that and still eat healthy.

It wasn't until I learned to prepare my food that I stepped into a body that's full of health and vitality that I love. A light bulb went off and I finally realized that the perfect meal wasn't just going to show up out there somewhere for me the way that I wanted it (and needed it) to be prepared. There were no readily available meals with the proper amount of protein, carbohydrates, starches, fiber, and good fats.

We are going to focus on a balanced diet with fresh ingredients and whole foods deliciously prepared. I want you to begin eating unafraid, without guilt, and learn to really get enjoyment out of your food. Food is our source of fuel and restoration. Truthfully, we can't survive without it so why not have a great relationship with it?

Cooking fresh food at home helps us steer clear of additives, preservatives, fillers, sodium, and emulsifiers that last on the shelf forever or keep your ice cream sandwiches from melting. I'm pretty sure if an ice cream sandwich won't melt out in the hot sun, ingesting it is only going to clog your arteries and wreak havoc on your health.

If you have been eating salty, overly sweet things, excessive sodium, and/or heavily spiced types of foods, it's going to take a while to adjust to the taste of natural food. Also, if you've mainly been grabbing food on-the-go, this will be hard for you at first. It's going to be a big change because you're used to convenience and not having to think about your food prep. Give yourself some time and grace to make the change. You have over 200 taste buds in your mouth so, in actuality, you can train yourself to like just about anything if you're hungry enough. I want you to retrain your brain to think of food as energy, not fat. We can have good energy or bad energy. The kind of energy we get from good fat will last a while and keep us satisfied. The kind of energy we get from eating a bowl of sugary cereal won't sustain us. We'll get a quick burst of energy but then it will die out and cravings will begin. I know many of you may be thinking, "But I don't like butternut squash or vegetables." You need to stop dwelling on what you don't like. Arnold Schwarzenegger said, "If it tastes good, spit it out." Now, I wouldn't go quite that far because there are so many ways to make your food fun, healthy, and delicious. Instead of using a condiment to liven up your food such as sugary ketchup or barbecue sauce, try using different types of mustard. They are low calorie, low sugar, low glycemic, and come in a great variety of spice.

Clean, unprocessed foods are much more calorie dense. When you have five egg whites for breakfast, they are around a total of 82 calories, which is much less than when you have a bowl of cereal with milk and its 200 calories. To build and maintain lean muscle, we need to focus on foods that provide good energy, such as egg whites. Really, basic nutrition is simple. Just eat real, whole, unprocessed foods. People like to over complicate things. Sharon Polsky, WBFF pro says, "The issue is the fitness industry. People want to make money and have to make you feel like nutrition is complicated to sell you the next best gimmick. If a program is so complicated that you can't get it right then it's not a successful program. Just eat real food."

Get the Metabolic Fires Burning

One of the biggest complaints I get from people that have a hard time losing weight is that their metabolism is stagnant. They're not hungry in the morning and they are generally not hungry until one in the afternoon. That is a sign that their metabolic fire is not burning. One of the worst things that you can do is to go almost all day without eating because then you're going to eat a lot at night when you're not able to burn calories back off. This compounds the problem—gaining weight and being unable to get it off. The first thing you need to do when your metabolism is slowed down is to get on a schedule. Eat first thing in the morning and then every three to four hours after that, regardless of hunger. Yes, that's right, I want you to eat when you're not hungry. When you eat when you're not hungry, a funny thing happens—you don't overeat. Give your body a balance of what it needs—proteins, veggies, carbohydrates, and good fats. I want you to work with your body. Eat when you're going to use carbohydrates and fat as fuel and make your body work for you. Work with your body, not against it. Preparation will be the key.

1. Eat first thing in the morning, even if you're not hungry. This will reset your metabolic clock and put you on a schedule, just like a baby.

    When you can go without breakfast and almost until lunch without eating, it isn't a good sign. It means you have a sluggish metabolism and you're not burning off your food very quickly. To lose weight, you need to get your body to use your food as fuel, just like how a car's engine uses gas and runs out. I want to give you just the right amount of gas to get you to the next meal, and then gas up again, and so forth. I want you to burn off your gas, not store it in your body.

2. Eat every three to four hours whether you're hungry or not. If you eat when you're not hungry on a regular schedule, then you won't overeat. Nighttime overeating problem solved.

One of the biggest complaints I get is people like to eat a lot at night and feel out of control with their eating. This is a major problem area for many people and a big reason why they're not seeing results. The Sisterhood of S.W.E.A.T. way to eat is throughout the day, fueling our bodies as they need it with a balanced plan that takes care of the urge to overeat and keeps food cravings at bay. We will eat every three to four hours, making sure to have a good carb or good fat which will keep our blood sugar from dropping. When you go without eating and your blood sugar drops, it immediately sets you up for cravings. Also, when you have too much sugar it spikes your insulin level, setting you up for a crash and burn later which creates cravings and causes your body to store fat.

When we go without eating for too long in the day, it sets us up for problems at night such as eating too much of the wrong types of foods all at once or snacking before bed when we're not going to burn it off. The best scenario is to spread out our calorie intake all throughout the day when we will burn it off and use it as fuel.

3.   Drink before you're thirsty. Begin drinking water early in the morning and all throughout the day. Drink one gallon per hundred pounds of body weight.

Drinking water helps keep us full and boosts our metabolism. Many studies have shown that drinking water before a meal helps with weight loss. I think a big reason for this is that a lot of times we mistake thirst for hunger. So just like I want you to eat before you're hungry, I want you to drink before you're thirsty. Drinking plenty of water prevents constipation and flushes out waste. Elimination is important to weight loss and overall health. Make sure you are drinking good clean, filtered water. Much of our water supply is contaminated with microbes, pesticides, plastics, metals, chlorine, fluoride (yes fluoride) and other toxins. So drinking tap water is less than ideal.

4. Eat one to two cups of steamed or raw veggies with every meal.

    Fibrous vegetable carbs - Fill up on fresh, bright, and colorful veggies. You get so many micronutrients, antioxidants, and fiber in every bite. Vegetables are an example of calorie dense foods that are full of fiber and will make you full. You can have your fill of vegetables without the fear of putting on the pounds. Vegetables also may protect you against certain types of cancer, reduce your risk of heart disease, diabetes and obesity. I know we all think of mashed potatoes, ice cream, warm bread, and macaroni and cheese as comfort foods. It might surprise you to know that vegetables can actually act as comfort foods in your body by lowering your cortisol and stress levels. Vegetables are loaded with B vitamins, magnesium, potassium, vitamin C, vitamin K and omega-3 fats which all play a role in relieving stress and giving you a foundation for greater overall health (Mercola).

5. Eat a protein the size of your fist at every meal.

    Protein - Protein boosts metabolism by stimulating thyroid function, has a blood sugar stabilizing effect, provides glutathione to the liver as a premiere antioxidant, assists lean muscle mass development, provides energy, and is a natural appetite suppressant. Even if you don't feel hungry, eat your protein. This will keep your metabolic furnace stoked and burning throughout the day as well as balance blood sugar levels. When you have cravings, try eating your protein first and watch your cravings disappear.

    When you eat enough protein you will typically eat fewer calories. Protein is very filling and causes you to feel satisfied. It takes two times the amount of calories to burn off protein than it does carbs and fats because protein is harder to digest. Protein will also help you retain your lean muscle mass. The more muscle you have, the more calories you burn at rest when you're sitting, sleeping, walking, or eating.

6. Keep your blood sugar from dropping by having a clean carb with your first two meals and a good fat the last two meals.

Carbohydrates - In the last few years there has been this whole high protein, low carb dieting trend and it has taken more than it's given. In order to be able to work out and be in a good mood, you need carbohydrates. Carbs are the building blocks for muscle. In order to build muscle, you need have to have energy to work out. In fact, you may get lean from just eating protein all the time but your skin will have a sunken in look. Carbohydrates fill out your muscle.

Now, I'm talking clean carbohydrates, not sugar enriched carbs. I'm not a fan of "If It Fits Your Macros" (IIFYM). The premise behind IIFYM is that if you have the appropriate ratio of protein, fat and carbohydrates that you can eat whatever you want as long as it fits that ratio. So if you have 100 calories of Oreos or 100 calories of an apple, supposedly that's the same. Now, this philosophy isn't taking into account what a fresh apple is going to do for me versus a ton of sugar and chocolate rushing around in my bloodstream. The types of carbohydrates we will focus on in the Sisterhood of S.W.E.A.T. are fresh fruits, vegetables, starches, fiber, and whole grains. Low glycemic carbohydrates won't spike your insulin levels like sugary carbs will. When insulin levels are spiked, fat will store more readily. The more sugary carbs you eat, the more belly fat you store. When I say sugary carbs I'm not just talking about candy. I'm talking about white bread, pasta, white rice, wheat bread, tortillas, and bagels that all turn into sugar within seconds in your mouth. Eating a balance of protein and fat would slow this process down significantly. Complex carbohydrates such as sweet potato, quinoa, brown rice, apples, and oatmeal will slow down the absorption of sugar thus providing more sustained energy throughout the day. The other problem with eating something sugary is that it will spike your insulin levels, giving you immediate energy but then you suffer a crash afterwards. This will cause you to have stronger cravings because as soon as your insulin levels spike and then come crashing down, you want more sugar. When you drink too much alcohol, have too much sugar, or have a history of taking antibiotics, you can also have yeast overgrowth. Candida albicans gobble up all the sugar in your gut which causes you to crave sugar. Another symptom of yeast overgrowth beside sugar cravings is recurrent yeast infections and sinus infections. When you have to take course after course of antibiotics, it also disturbs the good bacteria in your gut. I recommend taking a good probiotic whenever you take antibiotics to help prevent yeast infections. When you begin to connect the dots, you can see how all this connects. Consuming too much sugar is a vicious cycle.

7. Take in at least two tablespoons of good fat daily.

Eat Good Fats - Taking in good fat will decrease plaque in your arteries, raise good HDL cholesterol, and lower bad LDL cholesterol. According to research, you will even store less belly fat when you're taking in good fats (Mehmet). You can find good fat in olive oil and olives, canola oil, almonds, cashews, peanuts, nut butters, sesame seeds, and avocados. When you eat too many bad fats it keeps you from absorbing the good ones. Bad fats are in things like French fries, doughnuts, chips and fried chicken. So when you eat an overload of that type of food it's going to keep you from absorbing good fats. The brain depends on essential fatty acids to function so if you don't take them in, you won't have them available for brain function because the body doesn't naturally manufacture them.

Take one tablespoon of Essential Oils two times daily such as avocado, olive, Udo's, MCT, coconut, macadamia nut, and flaxseed or fish oil. Healthy fats actually aid in weight loss and encourage healthy bowel movements. Take in good fats to lose fat. Good fats will provide energy and you won't store them as belly fat. You can take your healthy fat in various ways:

1. Make a yummy salad dressing.

2. Put in a protein shake.
3. Mix in oatmeal or mashed sweet potatoes.
4. Put it on your meat to keep from being dry.

*Don't heat flaxseed or fish oil because they will lose their nutritional properties and please remember to keep them refrigerated. Avoid taking flaxseeds or psyllium husks within one to two hours of taking any medication. They may interfere with absorption of medication. Please check with your doctor if you are taking medication.

It's very important that you make sure to eat every three to four hours if you want to diminish cravings. Keep your diet balanced and don't miss any food group on the plan. Just because you don't feel like eating a clean carbohydrate or good fat doesn't mean you shouldn't. We are trying to create a stable environment for your metabolism. Just like you create a schedule for a baby, you need to have a base in order to build a good metabolism.

Kick Sugar Cravings to the Curb

Sugar is the devil.

Did you know that sugar is very addictive? The best way to get rid of sugar cravings is to not eat sugar. According to Dr. Mark Hyman, "Some animal studies show that sugar is eight times more addictive than cocaine" (Pesce). I repeat, the best way to eliminate sugar is to not eat it. In the Sisterhood of S.W.E.A.T., we will incorporate a good carbohydrate or a good fat every three to four hours to keep your blood sugar stable and steady. This will create less shifts in your insulin level therefore diminishing cravings. When you are giving up sugar it is even more important to have good clean carbohydrates as a replacement for the sugar your body has been getting on a daily basis. You may actually have some withdrawal symptoms depending on how much of the addictive white powder you've been taking in. You also need to learn to recognize what your hidden sugar sources are. For starters, white bread, wheat bread, pasta, and white potatoes are all just like putting sugar directly into your bloodstream. I know we all think we're doing better when we get wheat bread instead of white, but I hate to break it to you that just eating two slices of whole wheat bread will raise your blood sugar levels more than eating two tablespoons of sugar.

Eating excess sugar gives you a fatty liver. According to a Danish study which involved forty-seven people, one liter of sweetened drinks a day for a period of six months can produce up to twice the amount of average fat in the liver and abdomen (Aller et al.). The American Journal of Clinical Nutrition scientists concluded that people who drink more sweetened beverages dramatically increase accumulation of fat in their liver, which can lead to diabetes and cirrhosis (Maersk et al.).

Taking in good fats is one of the best ways to stave off sugar cravings. (I notice on days that I don't eat enough fat that I am ravenous and want to eat a lot of carbs.) According to researchers out of Bordeaux University, sugar set off reward signals in the brains of the mice they tested it on. The mice in the study worked way harder for sugar than any other substance (Bennett). What can we learn about ourselves from these mice?

Including L-glutamine & chromium in your supplement regimen will help to reduce sugar cravings. According to Dr. Julia Ross, author of *The Diet Cure*, "Willpower may not be the problem. You could be lacking or deficient in these key nutrients. Chromium helps people with blood sugar regulation issues and lowers insulin resistance which helps supply cells with glucose. Take 200 mcg of chromium with breakfast, lunch, dinner, and at bedtime" (Ross).

Glutamine can put a stop to even the most powerful sugar craving within minutes. Glutamine is an amino acid and natural food substance. Glutamine stops sugar cravings because it can be substituted for glucose in the Krebs cycle. Take 500-1500 mg of L-glutamine first thing in the morning, mid-morning, and mid-afternoon.

Glutamine and chromium aren't to be taken if you suffer from diabetes unless your doctor permits it.

Don't eat sugar spiking substances such as white bread, white flour, white rice/pasta, over processed foods, or high fructose corn syrup. Sugar includes corn syrup, maltose, lactose, fructose, sucrose, brown sugar, honey, and molasses. Don't be fooled by advertising ploys like "fat free cookies" (these are loaded with sugar). A big reason to stay away from these overly processed foods is that they have been stripped of all the good fiber which would've slowed down insulin response.

A Few Facts About Dairy

Chinese women get half the calcium of American women yet they have a much lower rate of osteoporosis (Lang). Drinking milk doesn't necessarily guarantee you will store calcium in your bones. Although we are the biggest milk drinking country, we also have the highest incidence of osteoporosis. In the Sisterhood of S.W.E.A.T, we consume very little dairy and try to get the majority of our calcium from other sources. Some other things to consider about dairy are: A calf grows to a cow on milk in 3-6 months. In this instance, milk is used to add weight very quickly. Also, many people are lactose intolerant or have a food allergy to milk—a symptom of which can be unwanted weight gain. You can get your calcium through other healthy sources too such as leafy greens, almonds, and salmon. Excellent healthy alternatives to milk are almond, rice, and coconut milk.

Wheat Isn't Really Even Wheat These Days

Wheat isn't the same these days compared to what our grandparents had down on the farm. In order to be mass produced, most wheat is being crossbred which has caused a significant change in its amino acid base. This has led to a large increase in the amount of celiac disease. These changes have been extremely hard on the human digestive system. Not to mention that by the time most wheat reaches you in the form of bread or pasta, it has been stripped of everything good. Normally, wheat's natural fiber would slow down an insulin spike. In the world we live in today, the mainstream marketplace is a fast paced and overly processed food environment. We should all take note if something says "enriched" because what it really should say is "stripped of all healthy benefits."

Eating a Gluten-Free Diet Doesn't Make You Automatically Skinny

When you go completely gluten-free, grains and items that are high on the glycemic index will react in your body just like having sugar does. So yes, cutting back on gluten is important if you're gluten sensitive and weight loss is your goal. Keep in mind though that it is important to cut back on the high carbohydrate content in gluten-free products. Also, beware when something is labeled "sugar-free" because that means there's probably a whole host of artificial sweeteners in there that are worse for you than any sugar ever was. I think we've established by now that sugar is not good for you. Anything that says in its marketing that it's free of something is almost sure to include something else you don't want to have. The label "fat-free" usually means it's sure to have tons of sugar in it which is what really adds fat to the body in the long run. "Sugar-free" claims will most likely have tons of artificial sweeteners included in them. It pays to read the label. When writing this book, I decided that it was important that whatever ingredients used in recipes were accessible and easy to find at the local grocery store or in the whole foods section. I didn't want readers having to search through the jungle and go a hundred miles to some certain store that might have the item I recommended. 90% of your choices make the difference. It's impossible to be perfect. Free yourself and live in the world of better choices. Don't underestimate yourself.

Eat Regularly - To keep cravings down we want to keep our blood sugar stable by eating regular low glycemic meals that won't spike insulin.

Go Cold Turkey - When you eat sugar, you want more sugar. To want sugar less, don't eat sugar! Go cold turkey and your cravings will diminish in 42-78 hours.

Eat Fruit - When you want something sweet, fruit is a good natural substitute. Low glycemic fruit such as blueberries, strawberries, raspberries, and Granny Smith apples won't spike your blood sugar.

Avoid Alcohol - Alcohol is generally loaded with sugar and will make your cravings worse.

Carbohydrates do raise blood glucose. To stabilize blood sugar, insulin must be released into the bloodstream. To decrease this occurrence, it is best to eat lower glycemic, low carbohydrate foods. The glycemic index is a great guide to let you know how high or low your foods are. A food being low on the glycemic index generally equates to lower carbs and lower calories with a few exceptions such as ice cream, mashed potatoes, and cheese. Carbohydrates with an index of 55 or below have slower absorption into the bloodstream and will sustain energy for longer, making them less likely to spike your insulin levels. This is what you want—to gain energy without storing fat. Carbohydrate portion sizes are also relative to managing glucose and blood sugar levels. Meats and fats don't have a GI because they do not contain carbohydrates. I have provided you with a basic glycemic index guide below.

Glycemic Index

Food	Average GI
Lettuce	10
Peppers	10
Mushrooms	10
Onions	10
Spinach	6
Broccoli	10
Tomato	6
Asparagus	8
Cabbage	6
Celery	0
Cauliflower	15
Cucumber	15
Kale	15
Turnips	30
White Potato (medium)	High 80s
Sweet Potato (medium)	61
Carrots (1/2 cup)	47
Butternut/Acorn Squash	50
Green Peas (1/2 cup)	48
Chick Peas (1 cup)	34
Green Beans	28
Parsnips	52
Cherries	22
Apple (medium)	38
Banana (medium)	56
Grapefruit	25
Grapes	46
Orange	43
Peach	42
Prunes	10

Cantaloupe	63
Plum	55
Raisins	28
Kiwi	52
Mango	51
Strawberry	49
Pineapple	66
Papaya	56
Watermelon	72
Pear	38
Dates	103
Oatmeal (not instant - 1/2 cup dry)	58
Brown Rice (1 cup long grain)	77
Whole Wheat Bread (1 slice)	71
Quinoa	53
Basmati	67
Couscous	65
Barley	28
Black Beans	30
Chickpeas	34
Navy Beans	31
Kidney Beans	29
Lentils	29
Cashews	27

Fat Cravings

Just like your body has sugar cravings, you might also have fat cravings. Fat cravings can be for milk, cream, ice cream, mashed potatoes, and cheese. Oh boy, these are the amazing comforts foods. When we eat these we are immediately comforted and feel great. Warm mashed potatoes are soothing to the soul. The reason behind this is that when we eat these, the reward hormone, dopamine, is released into the brain. This sensation creates a false high, making you want it again. You can be attracted to junk food, plain and simple, just because you're not eating real food.

Caffeine, Carbs, and Adrenals

A little caffeine is fine but when you have it in excess, it is very hard on the adrenals. The flight or fight response kicks in and adrenaline surges as a response to too much caffeine. Long-term overuse may burn out the adrenals so much so that you won't even feel any response from a caffeinated beverage. Generally, when someone that has been a caffeine addict cuts back for a week or two they began to notice more balanced energy levels throughout the day. Maintaining blood sugar balance is a function of the adrenal glands. When you have too much caffeine it causes your blood sugar to spike and then crash. This process really messes with your blood sugar. The response your body has is almost identical to having too much sugar. Sugar is also an adrenal stimulant, too much or too little really messes with your blood sugar and your adrenals (Lam). Good carbohydrates are needed to balance the blood sugar. So contrary to what you would think you need to eat, eat some good complex carbohydrates, but not in excess. In the Sisterhood of S.W.E.A.T., we will focus on keeping the blood sugar balanced. Though many times adrenal burnout can be labeled a thyroid problem because they're so similar in symptoms, their treatment should not be the same. I love coffee. The thing that I did not realize about coffee when I began writing this book is that you really want to get your coffee organic. Here is why—our coffee can be sprayed with over 240 possible pesticides. We get the majority of our coffee from developing countries that don't have stringent laws and use a variety of herbicides, fungicides, insecticides, and synthetic fertilizers, some of which are banned in the U.S. because they are so toxic. I am in love with Isagenix organic coffee. I can't believe the money I'm saving, how much better I feel, and how much trimmer my midsection has become since I started drinking organic.

Conquer Cravings

When you find yourself searching your cupboards, briefcase, and refrigerator for what you're craving, put your craving aside for five minutes and ask yourself these questions:

- Am I hungry?
- Is this what I want to eat?
- Is this what I want to eat now?
- Is there something else I could eat instead?
- Am I thirsty?
- What can I drink?
- Am I tired?
- Do I need to rest now?
- Am I upset?
- What's going on with me emotionally?
- How can I solve this with something other than food?
- (My personal favorite) Is this bringing me closer to my goals or further away?

Do any of these scenarios sound like you?

1. I'm really upset that someone has been attacking me at work and I am stressed out about it. Instead of talking to someone about it, I'm going to eat a bag of chips.
2. While I'm on the phone, I mindlessly begin snacking on a bag of pretzels.
3. I'm totally angry at my spouse but can't talk to him so I'm going to blow off steam by eating a pizza.

Tackle the problems that bother you instead of destroying yourself with food. I guarantee you that facing up and owning difficulties may seem scary in your mind but once you do, it will bring you a sense of relief and release. When we let go, we begin to shed the things we don't need. Everything starts in the minds and our ability to conquer problems will help us to believe we can conquer weight loss. The weight you've been carrying may be just a symptom of the things you've been holding onto on the inside—unforgiveness, fear, rejection, doubt, anger, belief, hate, worry, stress, frustration, heartache, the list is endless. Make your own list of problems and feelings that you believe may be holding you back. Many times we eat for emotional reasons, not physical ones. That is why it is so important to know there is a deep correlation between the two. Freeing your mind and spirit of problems and things that bind you and literally weigh you down can be the key to weight loss. The only way to stop the vicious cycle of emotional eating is to get in touch with your feelings and to deal with your problems in a more productive way.

Do This

1. Eat every 3-4 hours
2. Have breakfast
3. Fill up with fiber
4. Eat clean carbs
5. Take in good fats
6. Have lean proteins with every meal
7. Drink enough water

Instead of Food, Reward Yourself With:

- Music
- A massage
- A small glass of wine
- A nice sit down dinner
- Yoga
- Shopping
- Exercise
- Two bites of what you're craving
- A nap
- Light a scented candle
- Take a bubble bath
- A pedicure

- A manicure
- Try a new tea and have it in a fancy cup
- A change of scenery
- Go do something fun
- Try something new
- Take a ten minute walk
- Get outside
- Practice deep breathing
- Meditate
- Have coffee with a friend

Know What Your Food Triggers Are

Nuts – Nuts are great for keeping on hand in case you miss a meal at work. Keep a stash of nuts handy so you can grab a handful to keep your blood sugar stable. You wouldn't want to eat too many handfuls of nuts because it doesn't take too long before you're at your caloric intake for the day. So that could be a food trigger that you want to stay away from. Another thing you can keep on hand is nut butter which is very satisfying and quenches your appetite pretty easily. Don't keep nut butter on hand if you tend to eat the whole jar. You just want to have a tablespoon or two per day.

Chips - One of the reasons I consider chips to be such a food trigger is the monosodium glutamate (MSG) that's in most potato chips. Almost every single chip on the market contains MSG, which makes you crave more. That's why you can't eat just one and usually end up eating more than just a single serving size. If you're craving a snack that's crunchy, try some of these healthy alternatives: sliced red peppers with guacamole dip, salted apple slices, or cauliflower with hummus.

Chocolate - There are a multitude of reasons why you crave chocolate. For starters, the taste and the orgasmic endorphins it sends off into your brain, maybe you have a lack of magnesium in your system, maybe you're eating too little protein, stress, or you need an energy boost and since it is a stimulant, you dive for a piece of chocolate. Many times, if there is MSG in your chocolate it will be labeled as one of the following: whole mix solids, whey, soy lecithin, or hydrolyzed to name a few.

MSG - Here is an ingredient list to notify you if there may be MSG lurking in your favorite foods: artificial flavoring, calcium caseinate, Ajinomoto, Annatto, citric acid, caramel coloring, fat substitutes, hydrolyzed product, mix solids, barley malt, natural flavors, naturally processed corn syrup, free glutamic acid, dextrose, dextrin, disodium guanylate, disodium inosinate, maltodextrin, torula yeast, Umami, smoke flavors, stuffing mix, table salt, or texturized protein. Chicken and turkey are usually injected with MSG while evaporated milk and canned tuna usually contain calcium caseinate. You will also need to look for possible MSG in these food items: canned broth, bouillon cubes, croutons, canned or frozen vegetables, fruit products, fruit juices, bread yeast, butter, candy, table salt, carrageenan, whey, tortillas, baked goods, and corn products. Almost all fast food has MSG in it.

Here are some tips for avoiding MSG in your food. They don't have to tell you if a product has MSG in it.

Watch out for MSG in:
1. Processed food
2. Overly salty items
3. Products with a huge list of ingredients
4. Health food items (Just because it's from a health food store doesn't mean it's healthy.)

Let's Check the Bull at the Door

You're not going to get in shape by putting in minimal effort, working out just a couple of times a week, or taking low key exercise classes that require no more effort than a glorified pottery class all while eating fast food throughout the week. If you're eating out four times a week or eating just one supersized meal, you need to run four to five miles a day just to offset that. Another myth

I want to debunk is the misconception that fast food is cheaper. Really, there's nothing fast about fast food (except perhaps fast food = fast death). You have to get ready, get in your car, drive to the fast food place, wait in line, drive home, and then finally sit down and eat. After a month or two of that you find that your clothes are no longer fitting the way you'd like and you have to spend a lot more time exercising just to burn off what you're putting in your mouth. Further down the road, you may start to suffer from lack of energy, health problems, high blood pressure, and heart disease. In addition, you may have to start taking some type of medication to lower your cholesterol. Before you know it, your insurance goes up and your medical bills start to roll in, all of which could have been prevented if you'd just discovered food prep instead of fast food. If you're like most American families you don't have time to run four to five miles a day and/or you may not be physically able to. The good news is that 75%-85% of your results come from what you put in your mouth. All the exercise in the world will make little difference if you are eating poorly. That is why in the Sisterhood of S.W.E.A.T. your workouts are going to be hard… in the kitchen. If you work full time, I want you to set aside time to go to the grocery store and to complete weekly food preparation.

10
Prep & Plan

Meal Prep Made Easy

Tools:

- Large crockpot
- Large George Foreman grill
- Ninja 1000 or food processor
- Large steamer
- Large non-stick kettle
- Large non-stick skillet
- BPA-free plastic containers

Cook and shop once a week. - Stay ahead of the game by doing all of your grocery shopping and meal prep for the week on Sunday. Grocery shopping and meal preparation will take about two hours total. For the sake of convenience, get a steamer, a crockpot, a large George Foreman grill, and a Ninja 1000. These tools will make it easier for you to eat healthy and to get your food prep done in minimal time.

Multitask and get an assembly line going. - You can literally make everything at once—your chicken cooking in the crockpot, your ground beef cooking on the George Foreman grill, your veggies steaming in the steamer, your sweet potatoes and butternut squash baking in the oven, and your grains such as quinoa, brown rice, and/or oatmeal in a pot on the stove. If you want to get all of the sodium out of your chicken and cook it quickly, boil or simmer all of it in water. This takes about twenty minutes if it's boneless.

Purchase organic fruits and vegetables that are already washed and chopped. - For steamed vegetables I generally buy bags or boxes of organic vegetables that are already washed and chopped so all I have to do is pop them in the steamer. For vegetables that you may throw into stews, soups, or stir-fry, use the Ninja 1000. The Ninja chops your veggies up in no time. Chop up all of your other raw veggies and place in baggies. Some time saver tricks for veggies are to use low sodium canned green beans and frozen broccoli. Use organic salad or spinach in a box that is triple washed. Sometimes I will I cut up mushrooms, asparagus, onions, and red, green, and yellow bell peppers (which are unlimited fat-free foods) with any lean meat and put a lid over top and simmer in a skillet. It really is easy to eat healthy and there is no reason to depend on fast food, especially when you get in the habit of doing things this way.

As far as fruit goes, I follow the dirty dozen list. I buy my apples and berries completely organic so they are free from pesticides which can be detrimental to your health. Generally, I make sure to wash them so they are ready to grab when I need them. Frozen berries work great for your fruit but make sure you read the ingredients and that they do not have any added sugar.

Tips for washing fruit: Fill your sink with cold water and add a cup of white vinegar. This cleans the fruit, kills any unwanted surface bacteria or other contaminants, and helps preserve the fruit so that it will last longer.

The Dirty Dozen (12 Most Contaminated)

- Peaches
- Apples
- Sweet Bell Peppers

- Celery
- Nectarines
- Strawberries
- Cherries
- Pears
- Grapes (imported)
- Spinach
- Lettuce
- Potatoes

12 Least Contaminated

- Onions
- Avocado
- Sweet Corn (frozen)
- Pineapples
- Mango
- Asparagus
- Sweet Peas (frozen)
- Kiwi
- Bananas
- Cabbage
- Broccoli
- Papaya

Stock the Pantry

Purge your pantry of processed foods with five or more ingredients. Get rid of anything with hydrogenated oils, added sugar, monosodium glutamate, artificial flavors, and/or sweeteners. Use the grocery list provided on meal prep day.

Clean Pantry Foods

- Good fats
- Healthy oils
- Grains

- Beans
- Nuts
- Low glycemic flours
- Glass jars
- Buy canned goods that are low in sodium, without harmful preservatives, as well as BPA and sulfate free.
- Apple Cider Vinegar
- Aluminum free baking powder
- Stevia
- Spices

Keep Refrigerator Organized

Rid yourself of anything that could sabotage your eating plan. Eliminate foods that have not been eaten in over a week, that have expired, or may be spoiled. Organize your refrigerator by putting things with a longer shelf life such as sweet potatoes, squash, and apples on the bottom. Place vegetables and fruits in the crisper. Put meats, frozen vegetables, and fruits in the freezer. Keep meat that you will be cooking on meal prep day on the bottom shelf in bags.

1. Eggs and egg white cartons - middle shelf
2. Coconut, almond milk, and beverages - top shelf
3. Dairy products, cottage cheese, yogurt - bottom shelf
4. Raw meat products - bottom shelf
5. Vegetables, in bags - crisper
6. Fruit - crisper (To help prevent mold, use recommended white vinegar wash.)
7. Packaged meat - cold meat drawer or bottom shelf (where it's cooler)
8. Butter, yogurt, or goat cheese - dairy keeper
9. Condiments - door

Make sure to choose clean carbs and things from the list that will both satisfy your appetite and provide you with tons of energy like sweet potatoes, butternut squash, oatmeal, brown rice, and quinoa. You can bake up your sweet potatoes and squash for the week so they are ready in the fridge.

Clean out your refrigerator, pantry, and cupboards. I want you to eat all fresh whole foods and to shop the outer aisle of the grocery store. We are going to stick to nothing overly processed with five ingredients or less. I want you to be able to understand what you're reading on food labels and to know what is in your food. Don't be fooled by marketing schemes such as "96% fat-free," "multigrain," "all natural," or "sugar-free."

Fat-Free - When you buy something that is 96% fat-free it could actually be 50% fat. Look at the label and see how many calories actually come from fat and how many calories per serving determine the fat percentage. If there are 100 calories per serving and 50 of those calories come from fat, the product contains 50% calories from fat. Once you understand the math, there is a huge difference between percentage of fat by weight and percentage of fat by calories. It is understandable that you would be confused and think that when something such as a turkey burger label says it's 96% fat-free, you assume it is healthier. This type of marketing is very deceptive. The most popular myth is the fat-free dessert. This type of dessert is actually more fattening because they took out the fat which would've slowed down the absorption of sugar. Sugar is what makes you store fat in the first place.

Multigrain - I buy cereal that says "multigrain" and think I'm eating healthy but as Holistic Health and Thyroid Expert, Andrea Beaman would say, "It's just crack in a box." In reality, the carbohydrates in a lot of cereals are off the charts and there is a ton of sugar in them so it doesn't really matter that they are multigrain because they're also overly sweet and overly processed.

All Natural - GMO products are frequently labeled as "all natural" because they come from plants. They come from plants that have been crossbred with fish DNA or who knows what. For the purpose of this book, we will call them Frankenplants. Another misconception is that all natural meat doesn't have antibiotics or added hormones. Many of the "all natural" products have high fructose corn syrup in them which is highly processed and not even close to natural. If a product says "natural flavors," it can contain any one of 100 different chemicals, none of which are good for you.

Sugar-Free - Artificial sweeteners are laden with chemicals and are actually more addictive than sugar, if you can believe that. People drink twice the amount of soda than they would normally drink when it is a diet drink. Because artificial sweeteners are so much sweeter, they may cause you to think foods such as fruit aren't as appealing in taste. According to the Multiethnic Study of Atherosclerosis, drinking diet drinks daily was associated with a 36% greater risk for metabolic syndrome and a 67% increased risk for type II diabetes (Nettleton et al.). The bottom line is that you can't fool your body. Though artificial sweeteners are lower in calories, they trigger a lot of the same reactions that sugar does.

Artificial Sweeteners - When people are dieting, a lot of times they think, "I will have that diet soda instead of the regular soda with all that sugar. That's better, right?" Research shows that artificial sweeteners with aspartame, phenylalanine, sucralose and saccharin can all cause you to crave sweets (Yang). Although you may be having an artificial sweetener, your body will still treat it like sugar. The same physical reactions and bloating can occur. I can't believe I'm saying this but a little sugar is probably better for you than all of those chemicals.

Other Items to Watch out for Include:

- GMOs
- Trans fats
- Preservatives
- Refined sugars
- Nitrates
- Food dye
- Carrageenan
- Dough conditioners

Not All Fish Are Created Equal

I turned to a fitness expert that was on the cover of a well-known fitness magazine.

"Eat fish," the fitness expert said. "Eat fish morning, noon, and night. Eat fish until you get lean." That was the motto.

The problem with that was that they didn't tell me what type of fish to eat. No discussion about mercury poisoning or other side effects from a possible wrong choice was ever brought up. I could not for the life of me figure out why I was so exhausted after a full night sleep. At first I thought it was because I was doing fitness competitions, that it was the training, or maybe it was the diet. It couldn't be the diet, I thought, "I'm eating everything healthy!" Just because it's fish, doesn't mean it's healthy. I learned the hard way that not all fish are created equal. Here is the list I wish I had before I was diagnosed with mercury poisoning. You know what they say, hindsight is always better than foresight.

Low mercury
1. Fresh Salmon
2. Shrimp
3. Pacific Sole
4. Wild Tilapia
5. Anchovies

Moderate Mercury
1. Canned Tuna
2. Mahi-Mahi
3. Lobster
4. Halibut
5. Striped Bass

High Mercury
1. King Mackerel

2. Shark
3. Ahi Tuna
4. Swordfish
5. Marlin

Go with fresh, wild caught fish whenever possible. Some of the problems with farm raised fish are that they have high concentrations of antibiotics and pesticides, chicken feces is commonly one of the main ingredients in farm fish feed, they contain ten times the amount of cancer causing pollutants compared to wild fish, and their omega-3 levels may be reduced by as much as 50%. Seven out of ten fish are contaminated with PCBs which increase your risk of cancer and are usually raised in closed conditions, which breed sea lice, parasites, and disease.

A study from Wake Forest University found that the inflammatory potential farm raised tilapia is far greater than that of hamburger or bacon (Axe).

"Lack of activity destroys the good condition of every human being, while movement and methodical physical exercise save it and preserve it." ~Plato

Food Plan/Grocery List

P - Proteins
V - Vegetables
F - Fruits
C - Carbs
GF - Good Fats

P - Proteins
  Eggs
  Chicken Breast
  99% Lean Ground Turkey
  Canned Tuna in Water
  96% Lean Ground Beef
  Bison

White Fish
Wild Tilapia
Flounder
Cod
Salmon
Flank Steak
Shrimp

V - Vegetables

Broccoli
Cauliflower
Green Beans (low sodium)
Asparagus
Carrots
Celery
Cucumbers
Kale
Spinach
Romaine
Arugula
Mushrooms
Bell Peppers
Onions
Butternut Squash

F - Fruits

Berries (unsweetened)
Grapefruit
Apple
Lemon
Higher Glycemic Fruits
Banana
Grapes
Melon

Watermelon

Pineapple

Pears

Plums

Peaches

Orange

Nectarines

Kiwi

Pomegranate

C - Carbs

Brown Rice

Quinoa

Yams

Sweet Potatoes

Spaghetti Squash

Turnip

Zucchini

Tomatoes

Beets

Canned Pumpkin

GF - Good Fats

Almonds

Walnuts

Pecans

Cashews

Avocado

Flaxseed

Pumpkin Seed

Olive Oil

Coconut Oil

Udo's Oil

Flax Oil

Condiments:
Mustard
Balsamic Vinegar
Spices without sodium

Low Glycemic Sweeteners:
Stevia
Coconut Palm Sugar
Xylitol

Protein takes two to three hours to digest, fats take three to four hours, and carbs only take about forty-five minutes. Once food leaves your stomach, your brain automatically begins to give you signals that you're hungry again! You'll notice while on the Basic Meal Plan that you will stay full and satisfied longer! The nutrients and combination of foods in this plan are more filling, full of fiber, and have fewer calories. An apple alone is not a good breakfast choice and pretzels are not a good snack choice.

This is your whole foods clean eating chart. The letters in the chart correlate to the food group in The Basic Lifestyle Plan.

An example day might go something like this:

Meal 1 **P** - 4 ounces egg whites, **F** - ½ cup blueberries, **C** - ¼ cup quinoa

Meal 2 **P** - 4 ounces IsaPro, **F**- ¼ apple, sliced, **C** - 1/4 cup oatmeal

Meal 3 **P** - 4 ounces bison, **V** - 1 cup broccoli, **C** - ¼ cup couscous, **GF** - 1 tablespoon coconut oil

Meal 4 **P** - 4 ounces chicken breast, **V** - 2 cups romaine lettuce, **C** - ¼ cup quinoa, **GF** - 1 tablespoon olive oil (ACV salad dressing)

Meal 5 **P** - 4 ounces wild Alaskan cod, **V** - 1 cup asparagus, **GF** - ¼ cup slivered almonds

Meal 6 **P** - 4 ounces salmon, **V** - 1 cup Brussels sprouts, **GF** - almonds, handful

The Basic Plan Chart

Each letter stands for a food group and may be used as a reference for all plans in the Sisterhood of S.W.E.A.T.

The serving size amounts listed below are guidelines for the Basic Plan only and will vary according to your individual plan.

Proteins 4 ounces (Measure before cooking)	Vegetables 1-2 Cups	Fruits ½ Cup	Carbs ¼ Cup	Fats 1 Tablespoon
P	V	F	C	GF
Canned Tuna in Water	Cauliflower	Blueberries	Brown Rice	Almonds, Handful
96% Lean Ground Beef	Green Beans	Raspberries	Quinoa	Walnuts, Handful
Bison	(low sodium)	Strawberries	Couscous	Pecans, Handful
99% Lean Ground Turkey	Asparagus	Lemon/Limes	Millet	Cashews, Handful
Omega-3 Eggs	Scallions/ Green Onions	Apples	Oats	Avocado
Egg Whites	Celery	**Higher Glycemic Fruits**	Barley	Flaxseed
Chicken Breast	Cucumbers	Grapes	Brown Rice Flour	Pumpkin Seed
White Fish	Water Chestnuts	Banana	Quinoa Flour	Sesame Seed
Halibut	Kale	Strawberries	Rye Flour	Sunflower Seed
Chicken Breast	Spinach	Melon	Coconut Flour	Sesame Seed
Lamb	Romaine	Watermelon	Almond Flour	Flax Oil
Venison	Chard	Pineapple	Ezekiel Bread	Avocado Oil
Cod	Arugula	Papaya	Ezekiel Tortillas	MCT Oil
IsaPro	Mushrooms	Watermelon	Canned Pumpkin	Udo's Oil
IsaLean Pro	Bell Peppers	Pears	Turnip	Olive Oil

Flank Steak	Onions	Plums	Butternut Squash	Flax Oil
Shrimp	Eggplant	Peaches	Spaghetti Squash	Coconut Oil
Sardines	Brussels Sprouts	Oranges	Sweet Potatoes	Tahini
Tilapia	Bok Choy	Nectarines	Yams	Almond Butter(no sugar/salt added)
Flounder	Bamboo Shoots	Honeydew	Beets	Peanut Butter (no sugar/salt added)
Salmon	Cabbage	Pomegranates	Plantains	Cashew Butter
	Yellow Squash	Prunes	Acorn Squash	
	Acorn Squash	Mangoes	Carrots	
	Jalapeno Peppers	Raisins		
	Okra	Pomegranates		
	Artichokes			
	Jicama			
	Sea Vegetables			
	Rutabaga			
	Okra			
	Snow/Snap Peas			
	Artichokes			
	Tomatoes			

The Basic Plan in a Nutshell

P.	3-4 ounces of lean, clean protein at every meal
V.	1-2 cups of veggies, 4-5 meals
F.	½ cup fruit daily before 6pm
C.	¼ cup clean carbs, 3-4 meals (No complex carbs after 6:00 pm.)
GF.	2 tablespoons good fat, meal 5 and 6

Vitamins: Multivitamin of your choice

P.	Proteins
V.	Vegetables
F.	Fruits
C.	Carbs
GF.	Good Fats

The Basic Plan - Lifestyle

This is a non-processed, whole foods plan and can be done on an on-going basis. We do not eliminate any food groups, use quick fixes, gimmicks, or overdose you on hundreds of supplements.

Monday-Saturday - Follow the Basic Plan.

Sunday Funday - This is a planned treat meal or healthy cheat day. You can eat foods on Sunday in any order you choose from the grocery list and have one treat meal of your choice.

Meal 1 (5 min after waking)
    P. 3-4 ounces lean protein
    C. ¼ cup clean carb
    F.V. ½ cup fruit or 1-2 cups vegetable

Meal 2 P. 3-4 ounces lean protein
    C. ¼ cup clean carb
    F.V. ½ cup fruit or 1-2 cups vegetable

Meal 3   **P.** 3-4 ounces lean protein
            C. ¼ cup clean carb
            V. 1-2 cups vegetables

Meal 4   **P.** 4 ounces lean protein
            C. ¼ cup clean carb
            V. 1-2 cups vegetable
            GF. 1 tablespoon good fat

Meal 5   **P.** 4 ounces lean protein
            V. 1-2 cups vegetable
            GF. 1 tablespoon good fat

Meal 6   **P.** 4 ounces lean protein
            V. 1-2 cups vegetable
            GF. 1 tablespoon good fat

The Basic Plan - Lifestyle Instructions

This is a lifestyle plan in which you eat whole foods. No food groups are eliminated. You can continually eat this way for life.

- No alcohol.
- Get 6-8 hours of sleep per night.
- Drink 1 gallon of water per day.
- Weigh and measure your food.
- No diet soda. I know that this is going to be the hard one for some people but you have to eliminate soda of any kind. This is very important. Diet soda causes cellulite, adhesions under the skin, water retention, and can diminish skin elasticity. A study that Dr. Mercola brings to light in his article, *Artificial Sweeteners -More Dangerous than You Ever Imagined*, shows how much artificial sweeteners and aspartame can cause you to be hungrier and crave sweets. Dr. Mercola also refers to diet soda appropriately as a "formaldehyde cocktail" (Mercola). The Bressler Report found that aspartame had been tested by faulty procedures with inaccurate results concerning tumors found in lab animals. In 1979, the FDA established a Public Board of Inquiry (PBOI) to rule on safety issues with aspartame, with the result

that NutraSweet would not receive final approval pending further investigation into its link to brain tumors in animals.

- Fish. Feel free to eat fish when you like but watch for mercury advisories.
- It is very important to take accountability photos and to fill out your food journal each week. Pictures are worth 1,000 words and will help you to have measurable results.
- The first week will be the toughest. Try to cut out all overpowering tasting foods this week so you can re-train your taste buds to taste and enjoy the natural taste of foods. (You will begin to enjoy all foods especially when your metabolism raises and you're hungry.)
- It is very important to eliminate junk and fill up on healthy foods this week.
- Shop clean. Don't keep foods in the house that you don't want to eat. You should have to leave your house for a treat.
- Do your food preparation for the week on Sunday Funday.
- Sunday Funday - This is a planned treat meal or healthy cheat day. You can eat foods on Sunday in any order you choose from the grocery list and have one treat meal of your choice.
- Before the initial phase of the diet, it is important to purge the kitchen of all junk food and eliminate sugar, high fructose corn syrup, hydrogenated fats, refined grains, alcohol, and to limit caffeine.
- Stevia, coconut palm sugar, coconut crystals, and monk fruit are the only sweeteners I recommend on the plan. They are all natural and low glycemic. Honey and agave are okay if used sparingly.

The Basic Plan - Carb and Fat Rotation- (High/Medium/Low)

I like to use the next part of the plan to overcome a set point. A set point is the weight your body likes to stay at and is comfortable with. When your body is at its set point, you may feel stuck, in a rut, at a standstill, or that your body has reached a plateau. Carbohydrates and fats will be varied to sustain energy. This will create metabolic confusion and may help to stimulate weight loss. It is a good idea to lower your activity levels on your lowest carb day.

Plan to do your harder workouts and H.I.I.T. training on your high carb days and moderate workouts and steady state cardio on your medium days. Though your low days provide good fats, it is a good idea to lower your activity levels on your lowest carb day. What most people don't realize is that vegetables are also carbohydrates. Examples of starchy vegetables which are higher in carbohydrate content are corn, peas, parsnips, potatoes, pumpkin, squash, zucchini and yams. Non-starchy vegetables, lower in carbohydrates are typically flowering parts of the plant such as lettuce, asparagus, broccoli, cauliflower, cucumber, spinach, mushrooms, onions, peppers, and tomatoes.

Basic Plan - Carb and Fat Rotation
(Plan Length: 4-6 weeks)

Day 1 (High) - 2 carbs, 2 fats
Day 2 (Medium)1 carb, 3 fats
Day 3 (High) - 2 carbs, 2 fats
Day 4 (Low) - 0 carbs, 4 fats
Day 5 (High) - 2 carbs, 2 fats
Day 6 (Medium) - 1 carb, 3 fats
Day 7 (Low) - 0 carbs, 4 fats

What the plan looks like laid out:

High Rotation - Day 1, Day 3, & Day 5

Meal 1 (5 min after waking)
   P. 3-4 ounces lean protein
   C. ¼ cup clean carb
   F.V. ½ cup fruit or 1-2 cups vegetable
Meal 2 **P.** 3-4 ounces lean protein
   C. ¼ cup clean carb
   F.V. ½ cup fruit or 1-2 cups vegetable
Meal 3 **P.** 3-4 ounces lean protein
   V. 1-2 cups vegetable
   GF. 1 tablespoon good fat

Meal 4 **P.** 4 ounces lean protein
   V. 1-2 cups vegetable
   GF. 1 tablespoon good fat
Meal 5 **P.** 4 ounces lean protein
   V. 1-2 cups vegetable
Meal 6 **P.** 4 ounces lean protein
   V. 1-2 cups vegetable

Low Rotation - Days 4 & 7

Meals **P.** 3-4 ounces lean protein
1-4   **V.** 1-2 cups vegetable
   GF. 1 tablespoon good fat
Meals **P.** 4 ounces lean protein
5-6   **V.** 1-2 cups vegetable

Medium Rotation - Days 2 & 6

Meal 1   (5 min after waking)
   P. 3-4 ounces lean protein
   C. ¼ cup clean carb
   F.V. ½ cup fruit or 1-2 cups vegetable
Meal 2   **P.** 3-4 ounces lean protein
   F.V.. ½ cup fruit or 1-2 cups vegetable
Meal 3   **P.** 3-4 ounces lean protein
   V. 1-2 cups vegetable
   GF. 1 tablespoon good fat
Meal 4   **P.** 3-4 ounces lean protein
   V. 1-2 cups vegetable
   GF. 1 tablespoon good fat
Meals 5-6 **P.** 3-4 ounces lean protein
   V. 1-2 cups vegetable
   GF. 1 tablespoon good fat

Carb and Fat Rotation Instructions

- Eat every 3 hours, even when you're not hungry
- Have protein at every meal
- No alcohol or artificial sweeteners
- Get 6-8 hours of sleep per night
- Drink 1 gallon of water
- Fill out food journal
- Weigh and measure your food

Supplement Benefits

1. HCl – digestion
2. Probiotics – weight loss, energy, digestion
3. Apple cider vinegar – elimination, digestion, arthritis, belly fat
4. Coconut oil – thyroid healing, elimination
5. Maca (superfood) – energy, hormone balancing, antioxidant
6. Ashwagandha – stress, energy
7. Water – energy, recovery
8. Isagenix – organic meal replacement

7 Plateau Busters

When you have hit a plateau on the Basic Plan or the Basic Carb Rotation Plan, try some of these remedies. You can incorporate one or all five to get past your set point.

1. Drink ½-1 gallon of water daily.
2. Have 2 tablespoons of apple cider vinegar before meals with protein. (Please dilute with water or use as a salad dressing.)
3. Drink the slimming lemonade. It can be used as part of your water intake.
4. Eat 1 Flourless Muffin page 142.
5. Take 1 tablespoon of Slenderizing Oil two times daily.
6. Eat your protein.
7. Sleepy Night Cocktail (Get 7-8 hours of uninterrupted sleep.)

Belly Buster Tips

Banish Belly Fat!

Bloat Be Gone - Clean out metabolism downers such as beer, pizza, sugary carbs, yeasty white bread, and overly processed foods loaded with chemicals. Sugary or high glycemic carbs cause insulin, a fat promoting hormone, to be released into the blood. Beware of the "great whites"—cut out "white death" such as sugar and white flour and limit salt intake. This also includes all types of high insulin spiking foods made from the "great whites" such as pasta, pastries, rice, bread, cereal, crackers, and baked goods.

Protein - Even if you don't feel hungry, eat your protein. This will keep your metabolic furnace stoked and burning throughout the day as well as balance blood sugar levels. If you have cravings, always eat your protein first and then watch your cravings subside. Not all protein powders are created equal. Protein powder boosts metabolism by stimulating thyroid function, stabilizing blood sugar, providing glutathione (the liver's premiere antioxidant), assisting in lean muscle mass development, and providing energy. It is also a natural appetite suppressant. Try to choose one sweetened with Stevia which keeps the insulin level down.

Drink Water

Apple Cider Vinegar - I swear by apple cider vinegar and incorporate it every day. Since beginning the ACV regimen, I have personally noticed a significant difference in my mid-section. The reason for this is that ACV promotes health and weight loss by aiding digestion and elimination. ACV also contains potassium, pectin, and calcium. ACV helps to maintain healthy pH levels. It will enable your body to break down fats and use them for energy instead of storing them. To help banish belly bloat, take it before each meal. Dilute in water. Use unfiltered apple cider vinegar with the mother in it. The mother is the best part of the apple and is left out of many store bought brands due to over-processing. Bragg's apple cider vinegar with the mother is easily found at your regular grocery store in the health food section. You can have it numerous different ways—in salad dressing, dilute it in water, or marinate your meat in it. I wouldn't recommend drinking it straight. Drinking ACV straight down undiluted can cause the gag reflex, burn your esophagus, close off your windpipe, and wreak havoc on the enamel of your teeth. I'm a big believer in this reducing the false fat you see around your middle that's caused by hanging on to toxic waste when the digestive system isn't operating at its fullest potential. For this, apple cider vinegar is one of nature's amazing gifts.

ACV Benefits

1. Helps with digestion.
2. Helps with process of elimination.
3. Relieves gout.
4. Helps reduce inflammation.
5. Reduces arthritis pain.
6. Lowers blood pressure.
7. Helps break down fat.
8. Help prevent the flu and stomach illness.
9. Clears fungus and bacterial rashes.
10. Helps to prevent acne, lowers blood sugar levels, and removes brown spots.
11. Helps with weight loss.
12. Some studies have shown ACV to shrink tumors and help kill cancer (Mimura et al.).

Flourless Muffin Ingredients

Ground Flaxseed - Flaxseed will fill you up and help to regulate bowels and balance hormones.

*Don't take any oils, flaxseed, or psyllium husks within one to two hours of taking any medication. They may interfere with absorption of medication.

Cinnamon - Cinnamon has antifungal, antibacterial, and anti-parasitic properties. Cinnamon has been found to be effective in fighting vaginal yeast infections, oral yeast infections, stomach ulcers, and helps to lower insulin levels and control blood sugar. Cinnamon is also a great source of manganese, fiber, iron, and calcium.

Omega-3 Eggs - Omega-3 eggs are loaded with sulfur and lecithin which aid the liver in the fat burning process. Benefits include improved brain function, focus, and relief for rheumatoid arthritis. Omega-3 eggs also inhibit overeating and reduce inflammation in the body.

Cacao Powder - The highest whole food source of magnesium, cacao powder dissolves plaque in the arteries and lowers blood pressure. Very high in antioxidants such as resveratrol and polyphenols, catechin and epicatechin, cacao also contains omega-6 fatty acids, tryptophan, and serotonin. This superfood also has chromium and coumarin content which helps with weight loss and regulates blood sugar (Kilgour).

Protein Powder - Protein powder boosts metabolism by stimulating thyroid function, stabilizing blood sugar, providing glutathione (the liver's premiere antioxidant), and assisting in lean muscle mass development. It also provides energy and is a natural appetite suppressant. Try to choose one sweetened with Stevia which keeps the insulin levels down.

Slenderizing Oils - Take one tablespoon of Slenderizing Essential Oils two times daily such as avocado, olive, coconut, macadamia nut, flaxseed, or fish oil. These healthy fats actually aid in weight loss and encourage healthy bowel movements. Take in good fats to lose fat. Good fats will provide energy and you won't store them as belly fat. You can take your healthy fat in various ways—make a yummy salad dressing, put in a protein shake, or mix in oatmeal or mashed sweet potatoes. Don't heat flaxseed or fish oil and remember to keep it refrigerated.

*Don't take any flaxseed or psyllium husks within one to two hours of taking any medication. They may interfere with absorption of medication.

Coconut Oil (The Tree of Life) - Coconut oil aids in weight loss, energy, is good for skin, hair, and the thyroid gland. It also contains antibacterial and antimicrobial properties (Mercola).

Take one tablespoon 1-2 times a day with meals. Coconut oil can also be used in salad dressings, sauces, or any type of cooking. It has a very mild taste and quickly melts in your mouth. Product solidifies at 78°F.

Coconut Oil Benefits

- Promotes weight loss
- Supports the thyroid
- Improves digestion and elimination
- Help prevent Alzheimer's
- Provides energy
- Antimicrobial
- Helps prevent hemorrhoids
- Kills bacteria
- Kills fungi and yeast
- Dissolves kidney stones
- Expels or kills tapeworms, lice, giardia, and other parasites
- Boosts energy and athletic performance
- Diminishes the appearance of stretch marks
- Great for your skin
- Protects the body from free radicals

Catch Some Zzzzz's!

Proper sleep is important! In a sixteen year study of over 70,000 middle-aged women, those who got five or less hours of sleep were likely to experience a major weight gain of thirty-three pounds or more. Sleep deprived women are also more likely to become obese. According to the University of Chicago, lack of sleep creates cravings. If you sleep seven to eight hours a night, you secrete half as much cortisol as those who sleep six or less (Van Cauter et al.).

Sleepy Night Cocktail

Ingredients:
2 tablespoons tart cherry juice
2 tablespoons apple cider vinegar
Natural Vitality Natural Calm - follow directions for recommended dose on the bottle

Instructions:
Mix together tart cherry, Natural Calm, and ACV in a large mug with 8 ounces of water. The Calm will fizz up so don't pour in the water all at once. The tart cherry antioxidants combined with the apple cider vinegar's properties are helpful for arthritis and inflammation. The calm powder aids in better sleep, helps to balance calcium, and restores magnesium levels. Tart cherry juice's major attributes include combating gout, acting as a powerful inflammation fighter, and helping to reduce insomnia.

In a 2013 article in Osteoarthritis and Cartilage, researchers at the Philadelphia VA Medical Center found that "patients who drank two 8-ounce bottles of tart cherry juice daily for 6 weeks experienced a sizeable improvement in pain, stiffness, and overall physical function. The Study participants demonstrated a significant decrease in high sensitivity C-reactive protein (CRP), which is a marker of inflammation. Each bottle of juice is equivalent to approximately 45 cherries."

ACV is rich in beneficial enzymes and acids that aid in digestion and the absorption of nutrients which are crucial for joint health. The acetic and malic acid in ACV helps to detoxify the body by helping to eradicate toxins, waste, and restore the body's pH level.

Taking Natural Calm may help improve your sleep patterns. According to a study in the September 2001 issue of Behavior Genetics, "normal sleep patterns are linked with having sufficient levels of magnesium. In the study, levels of magnesium in the bodies and brains of rats were measured.

Researchers determined that rats that had more consistent sleep had higher levels of magnesium. Rats with lower magnesium suffered more abnormal sleep patterns" (Callahan).

11
The Recipes

Recipes

When you are deciding what to make, there are letters provided with each recipe that correspond to the Basic Plan Chart. To order your Isagenix products from the recipe section, go to http://lindalu7.isagenix.com/

P - Proteins
V - Vegetables
F - Fruits
C - Carbs
GF - Good Fats

Flourless Protein Muffin - P F GF

Yields 4 servings.

Ingredients:
¼ cup organic applesauce (unsweetened)

¼ cup organic blueberries

1/8 cup ground flax

1 teaspoon baking powder

1 teaspoon cinnamon

2 scoops chocolate IsaPro

2 teaspoons organic cacao powder

2 tablespoons coconut oil

3 tablespoons egg whites

¼ cup stevia

3-4 stevia packets or 3 tablespoons xylitol

Instructions:
1. Mix all ingredients together and bake at 350°F for 10 minutes.
2. Allow to cool to a safe temperature and enjoy!

Turkey Curry - P C GF

Ingredients:

1 pound ground turkey breast

1 organic red pepper

1 organic orange pepper

1 organic green pepper

1 organic onion

8 ounce organic tomato sauce (unsweetened)

1 tomato

¾ cup coconut milk (unsweetened)

Olive oil

1 teaspoon curry

1/8 teaspoon cayenne pepper

Instructions:

1. Dice up red, orange and green bell peppers. Cut up white or yellow onion.
2. Sauté veggies in heated pan on medium heat with olive oil. Let veggies get somewhat softer in texture but not mushy. Then, add in tomato sauce and one diced tomato.
3. In a separate pan, sauté ground turkey breast.
4. Add 3/4 cup of unsweetened almond milk and mix together.
5. Sprinkle curry, cayenne pepper (for spice), and tarragon to mix.
6. Add turkey meat to vegetable pan and let simmer on low for 2 minutes.

Curried Chicken Salad Sandwich - P V F GF

Ingredients:

4 boneless chicken breasts, cooked and shredded (meatless option - chickpeas)

1 teaspoon basil

2 teaspoons spicy mustard

¼ teaspoon cayenne pepper

½ teaspoon chili powder

1 teaspoon curry powder

1 avocado

½ cup organic celery, diced

2 tablespoons extra virgin olive oil

½ teaspoon sea salt

1/8 teaspoon ground black pepper

½ teaspoon garlic

1 tablespoon organic lemon juice

2 tablespoons red onion, diced

Instructions:

1. Place the cooked, shredded chicken in a medium sized mixing bowl.

2. Put the basil, avocado, celery, onion, olive oil, all of the spices, and garlic in a food processor or chop daddy and blend.

3. Pour the avocado and basil mixture into the mixing bowl with the shredded chicken. Add lemon juice and olive oil and toss together. (The lemon juice keeps the avocado from turning brown. This will keep in the refrigerator for about 2-3 days if covered!)

4. Use lettuce and make a wrap!

Cinnamon Apple Slice (Replace Sandwich Bread) P F V

Ingredients:
2-3 large crisp, sturdy apples
2 packets stevia
½ teaspoon cinnamon
1 purple onion, sliced
Curried chicken salad

Instructions:
1. Put your curried chicken salad on a cinnamon apple slice.
2. Core your apple and slice across the center to make an apple round. Use just like you would a slice of bread.
3. Slice all apple rounds about a quarter of an inch thick.
4. Roll apple slices in cinnamon and stevia mixture until lightly coated.
5. Put a piece of lettuce and a slice of purple onion on the apple round with ¼ cup of chicken salad mixture on top.

Makes 14-16 rounds.

Sweet Potato Shepherd's Pie - P V C GF

Ingredients:

Meat & Veggie Filling:

1 purple onion, diced

½ teaspoon garlic powder

1 pound grass-fed beef or ground turkey (meatless option - 3 cups cooked organic black beans)

1 bag of organic baby carrots, diced

2 organic celery stalks, diced

1½ cups organic broccoli, chopped

1½ cups organic cauliflower, grated or chopped

1 teaspoon pepper

½ teaspoon thyme

½ teaspoon rosemary, dried

½ teaspoon sea salt

¾ cup beef broth

2 tablespoons Glen Muir tomato paste

2 tablespoons refined olive oil or coconut oil for sautéing

Potato Topping:

3 medium organic sweet potatoes

¼ teaspoon garlic powder

1/8 to ¼ teaspoon cayenne

½ teaspoon rosemary

¼ cup coconut or almond milk (unsweetened)

1 tablespoon butter

Instructions:

1. Peel sweet potatoes and slice them into wedges using a large knife. Or boil the sweet potatoes with the skins on, let them cool, then peel the skins off easily, and mash them.

2. Boil the sweet potatoes in water for 20 minutes or until you can poke a fork through them and they are soft, not mushy.

3. Drain the water from the pan.

4. Mash the potatoes with butter and milk, add the spices, and beat with a mixer until stiff, yet creamy.

5. Sauté your meat, purple onion, broccoli, cauliflower, celery, and carrots in a skillet over medium-high heat about 10 minutes with 2 tablespoons olive oil or refined coconut oil.

6. Mix in spices and beef broth with the tomato paste.

7. Simmer together about 10 minutes. Make sure veggies are cooked and somewhat firm, but not mushy.

8. Put the meat mixture in a large baking pan and spread mashed potatoes evenly over the top.

9. Bake at 350°F for about 30 minutes.

If you're looking for a special recipe to prepare for company, this is definitely worthy. Freaking delicious.

Optional: Place the shepherd's pie in the oven on broil for a couple of minutes to get a golden brown hue. Make sure to keep an eye on the pie so you don't overcook it.

Pot Pie with Pumpkin Crust - P V C GF

Ingredients:

Crust:
1½ cups oat flour or Namaste gluten-free perfect blend (Costco)
2 teaspoons sage, dried
1 teaspoon aluminum-free baking powder
½ teaspoon sea salt
2 tablespoons olive oil
1½ cups fresh or canned pumpkin

Filling:
1 teaspoon olive oil
1 teaspoon sea salt
¼ teaspoon ground black pepper
¼ teaspoon paprika
1½ pound lean turkey or chicken breast
1 medium onion, diced
1 celery stalk, chopped
1 bag frozen peas and carrots
½ teaspoon garlic powder
10 ounces frozen sweet potato, chopped
3-4 tablespoons coconut or oat flour
2 tablespoons coconut oil
1 cup fat-free, low-sodium chicken broth
2 cups coconut milk
1 teaspoon rosemary, freshly chopped
Olive oil cooking spray

Crust Instructions:
1. Prepare crust in a large bowl—add one of the half cups flour, sage, baking powder, and salt.
2. Stir with a fork to combine. Stir in buttery spread until mixture is crumbly in bowl.

3. Use your hands to knead dough 5 to 6 times until dough clings together, is softened, and slightly sticky, about 1 min.
4. Do not overwork the dough. Refrigerate dough for 30 min.

For the Filling:

1. Slice up poultry on chopping board into bite-size pieces.
2. Heat oil to medium-high in a large saucepan. Throw in bite-size pieces of poultry, onions, sweet potatoes, celery, carrots, and sauté for 10 minutes.
3. To make sauce, we will prepare it like white sauce. Heat coconut oil until bubbly and mix in coconut flour until thick. Remove from heat and add your spices.
4. Place the white sauce mixture back onto the stove and let it get a little bit bubbly.
5. Add coconut milk and chicken broth, gradually stirring until well mixed.
6. Cook until mixture begins to thicken.
7. In a large sauté pan, brown turkey, salt, and pepper, to taste.
8. Mix all the ingredients together and place in a 13x9 pan.
9. Roll out the crust on nonstick wax paper or a nonstick pastry mat.
10. Put the dough on top of the filling and bake at 350°F for 30 to 40 minutes

Chicken Bok Choy – P V

Ingredients:

1 large bok choy, cleaned and chopped

1 pound organic chicken breast

1 large onion, diced

3 cups Imagine chicken broth (unsweetened)

Instructions:

1. Sauté chopped bok choy and large diced onion in olive oil until soft.

2. Cut up chicken into small bite-size pieces on chopping board and sauté in separate skillet spritzed with olive oil.

3. Put chicken into bok choy and onion mixture.

4. Pour in 3 cups of Imagine chicken broth (or more if you want to eat it more like a soup).

Sometimes I like to have it as a hot soup on a cold day and other times I like to serve it over cooked quinoa. This is a very versatile dish.

White Chili - P V C GF

Ingredients:

2 cans organic white beans

1 can organic cannellini beans

1 tablespoon olive oil

1 pound organic chicken breast

1 large onion, chopped

1 large red pepper, chopped and seeded

1 jalapeno, chopped and seeded

1 small can of chopped chilies

4 cups of Imagine chicken broth (unsweetened)

1 teaspoon sea salt

1/8 teaspoon ground black pepper

1 tablespoon cumin

1 teaspoon chili powder

¼ teaspoon garlic powder

Instructions:

1. Slice up chicken breasts on chopping board into bite-size pieces.
2. Chop up onion, red pepper, and jalapeno pepper.
3. Sauté chicken breast, red pepper, onion, and jalapeno in 1 tablespoon of olive oil.
4. Open beans, drain juice, and pour into large saucepan. Mix in seasonings, chilies, beans, and chicken broth.
5. Put the chicken, onion, and pepper mixture into the bean mixture and simmer on low for 20 minutes.

Pumpkin Cornbread - P C

Ingredients:

1 cup pumpkin

1 teaspoon cinnamon

½ teaspoon ginger

¼ teaspoon nutmeg

1/8 teaspoon cloves

1 cup Namaste Perfect Blend Gluten-Free Flour

1 cup coconut milk (unsweetened)

½ cup coconut palm sugar

1 tablespoon aluminum-free baking powder

1 cup Bob's Mill GMO-free cornmeal

2 organic omega-3 eggs

Instructions:

1. Preheat oven to 350°F.
2. Grease a 9x9 pan.
3. Mix together dry ingredients in a large bowl.
4. Blend wet ingredients together with the mixer.
5. Pour wet ingredients into dry ingredients and beat with a mixer until smooth and creamy. Add more coconut milk if it's too dry.
6. Bake 35 to 40 minutes or until golden brown on top.
7. Cool and cut into 16 squares.

Dena's Competition Patties - P C V

Ingredients:

1½ pounds lean ground turkey (99% fat-free)

1 tablespoon fresh cilantro

1 cup spinach or celery

¼ cup green onions, chopped

1 teaspoon garlic, crushed

1½ cup brown rice, cooked

Instructions:

1. In a bowl, mix all ingredients together, then add a little salt and pepper.
2. Make meat mixture into small patties on a cooking sheet.
3. Bake in the oven at 350°F for about 20 to 30 minutes.

This is a great healthy snack and full of protein.

Sweet Tater Chili - P V C GF

Ingredients:

2 tablespoons coconut oil

2 pounds your choice of lean meat:

ground beef, ground turkey, ground chicken, ground bison (meatless option -

2 15-ounce cans of organic pinto beans)

2 sweet potatoes, cubed

1 medium onion, chopped

½ red pepper, chopped

½ green pepper, chopped

3 zucchini, diced

3 yellow squash, diced

1 teaspoon garlic powder

1 jalapeno, eliminate seeds

2 tablespoons cumin

1 teaspoon cinnamon

1 tablespoon chili powder

½ teaspoon paprika powder

2 tablespoons organic tomato paste

2 15-ounce cans organic diced tomatoes

1 cup beef broth (my favorite is Kitchen Accomplice)

1 teaspoon sea salt

¼ teaspoon pepper

Instructions:

1. Sauté meat, onion, sweet potatoes, red pepper, green pepper, zucchini, yellow squash, and jalapeno on medium-low heat until meat is brown.

2. Put in all spices, salt, pepper, beef broth, diced tomato, optional pinto beans, and tomato paste and simmer 5 minutes on low heat

<u>Sweet Potato Hash - P V C GF</u>

Ingredients:

2 tablespoons coconut oil

1 pound of bison burger

½ cup purple onion, chopped

4 cups baby kale

1 large sweet potato, diced

1 tablespoon Kirkland's organic No-Salt Seasoning

Instructions:

1. Sauté bison, diced sweet potato, and chopped onion in 2 tablespoons of coconut oil on medium-low heat until the sweet potato is soft.
2. Add in the kale and seasonings.
3. Cook 5 minutes more or until it is to your liking.

Zucchini Pancake - P V C GF

Ingredients:

4 organic egg whites

1 organic omega-3 egg

¼ cup Chia seed

¼ cup purple onion, chopped

1 cup zucchini

1 teaspoon chili powder

1/8 teaspoon cayenne pepper

1 teaspoon cumin

1 teaspoon cilantro

1 teaspoon onion powder

¼ teaspoon garlic powder

1 teaspoon sea salt

2 slices avocado

Instructions:

1. Combine egg whites with one whole egg and beat. Mix in all spices.
2. Sauté shredded zucchini purple onion in the pan.
3. Add the eggs, pour them over the zucchini, cook like a pancake, and flip.
4. Serve with half a slice of avocado, salsa optional.

Breakfast Quiche - P V C GF

Quiche Crust:

Ingredients:
¼ cup black Chia seed
¼ cup water
1½ cups quinoa, cooked
1½ tablespoons avocado oil
2 tablespoons nutritional yeast
¼ teaspoon sea salt

Instructions:
1. Preheat the oven to 400°F.
2. Grease a 13x9 pan.
3. Combine the Chia seed, water, nutritional yeast, quinoa, avocado oil, and salt in a medium sized bowl. Let it set until it thickens.
4. Press the crust evenly into the bottom and sides of the 13x9 pan.
5. Bake for 12-15 minutes or until golden brown.
6. Turn down the oven to 350°F after the crust is done. Then, bake the quiche 30-40 minutes or until golden brown at 350°F.

Quiche Filling:

Ingredients:
1 tablespoon avocado oil
½ teaspoon onion powder
1 teaspoon garlic powder
2 bunches asparagus
1 purple onion
2 carrots, chopped
16 ounce carton organic egg whites
½ cup pumpkin
1 tablespoon lemon juice
2 tablespoons nutritional yeast
1 teaspoon sea salt

Dash of black pepper

2 teaspoons Dijon mustard

½ teaspoon turmeric

Instructions:

1. Skin and core your onion.
2. Chop the purple onion into quarters.
3. Rinse and chop your asparagus, breaking the ends off.
4. Clean your carrots.
5. Throw all of your vegetables into the ninja 1000 or your food processor and blend until smooth.
6. Toss your spices and remaining ingredients in, blend until well mixed.
7. Pour into your 13x9 pan.
8. Bake 30-40 minutes at 350°F or until golden brown.

Healthy Mac-n-Cheese - P F C

Ingredients:

2 tablespoons organic butter (unsalted)

¾ cup coconut milk (unsweetened)

1 cup organic pumpkin, cooked

1 tablespoon organic Santa Cruz lemon juice

5 ounces Oasis red pepper hummus (zero fat)

1½ tablespoons arrowroot powder

7 tablespoons nutritional yeast

2 teaspoons Dijon mustard

¾ teaspoon garlic powder

1 teaspoon onion powder

1 teaspoon sea salt

16 ounces quinoa elbow macaroni

Instructions:

1. Boil macaroni in a large pot according to the directions.
2. Make cheese sauce in another large pot.
3. Melt butter on low heat.
3. Mix nutritional yeast, arrowroot powder, salt, onion powder, and garlic powder into butter until thick and bubbly.
4. Pour in the coconut milk and stir until smooth with no lumps.
5. Stir sauce until it begins to thicken.
6. Mix in pumpkin, lemon juice, mustard, and hummus.
7. Drain and rinse macaroni.
8. Pour cheese sauce over top and mix together until well blended.

Gluten Free Tortillas - C GF

These are delicious for any time you're feeling like eating bread but don't want to have anything with the yeast, sugar, or gluten.

Yields about six 9-inch tortillas.

Ingredients:
2 cups Namaste Gluten-Free Perfect Flour Blend
1½ teaspoons sea salt
2 teaspoons baking powder
5 tablespoons grass-fed butter (unsalted), cold and cut into 1 tablespoon pieces
¾ cup hot water
Flour for rolling

Instructions:
1. Mix flour, salt, and baking powder together. Use a pastry cutter or a fork to blend in butter until it is a dry and crumbly mixture.
2. Pour in water and mix until dough clings together.
3. Divide dough evenly into 6-7 balls.
4. You can roll the dough out onto parchment paper with some flour or use a tortilla press.
5. Spray your skillet or tortilla press with Pam or coconut oil and heat to medium-high.
6. Cook tortillas on each side for 60 seconds or until they bubble.

Avocado spread - F GF

I like to use this spread for tortillas. Besides tasting delicious, it helps everything to stay put while making a wrap, making it less messy to eat.

Ingredients:
One large avocado
½ teaspoon chili powder
½ teaspoon garlic powder
½ teaspoon sea salt
¼ teaspoon cayenne pepper
1 tablespoon lemon juice

Instructions:
1. Mash avocado, add seasonings and lemon juice, mix well.

Guacamole - V F GF

If you must have crunch, this is a great snack to dip raw veggies in.

Ingredients:

2 cups avocado, mashed

1 large tomato, chopped

¼ white onion, diced

¼ cup fresh cilantro, chopped

¼ cup lime juice

2 fresh jalapeño chili peppers, minced

¾ teaspoon sea salt

Instructions:

1. Combine mashed avocado, chopped tomato, diced onion, fresh cilantro, lime juice, minced chili peppers, and salt in a medium bowl.
2. Stir until combined.
3. Serve immediately.

Serve with turnip fries, use as sandwich spread, or as a veggie dip.

<u>ACV Salad Dressing - GF</u>

Ingredients:

1 tablespoon olive oil

2 tablespoons apple cider vinegar

1-2 teaspoons spicy mustard

Instructions:

1. Mix all ingredients together with a whisk.
2. Add stevia to sweeten (optional).

Sweet Potato Pancakes - P C

Great fuel for an athletic event or race day.

Ingredients:

1¼ cups gluten-free oat flour

¼ cup pecans, chopped (optional)

2¼ teaspoons baking powder

1 teaspoon pumpkin pie spice

¼ teaspoon sea salt

1 cup coconut milk (unsweetened)

¼ cup stevia or coconut palm sugar

1 tablespoon coconut oil

1 teaspoon vanilla extract

2 eggs, lightly beaten

16 ounces sweet potatoes (¾ cup mashed and drained) or cooked pumpkin

Instructions:

1. Mix all ingredients together and beat with mixer.

2. Spray pan with oil and make your pancakes. You can have real maple syrup if desired.

Pumpkin Bread - P F C GF

Yields about 12 slices.

Ingredients:
Olive oil spray
2 cups Namaste Gluten-Free Perfect Flour Blend
1½ teaspoons baking powder
½ teaspoon baking soda
¼ teaspoon sea salt
2 teaspoons cinnamon
½ teaspoon ginger
½ teaspoon ground nutmeg
1/8 teaspoon ground cloves
½ cup organic egg whites
1 teaspoon pure vanilla
1½ cups canned pumpkin
¾ cup coconut crystals
¼ cup refined coconut oil
¼ cup organic applesauce (unsweetened)

Instructions:
1. Preheat oven to 350 degrees F.
2. Lightly coat a 9x5 loaf pan with olive oil spray.
3. In a medium bowl, stir together all dry ingredients.
4. In a large bowl, combine all wet pumpkin mixture ingredients.
5. With a spatula, fold all dry ingredients into pumpkin mixture until just combined. (Do not overmix.)
6. Bake for about 45 minutes or until a toothpick inserted into center of bread comes out clean.
7. Let cool in pan on a wire rack for 15 minutes. Remove to finish cooling.

Store bread in the refrigerator for up to 1 week or in the freezer for up to 2 months.

For an added treat, stir ½ cup (total) of blueberries, chopped walnuts, almonds or cacao nibs into batter before spooning into pan.

Sweet potato chips - C GF

Ingredients:

3 large organic sweet potatoes

2 tablespoons refined coconut oil or pure olive oil

¼ cup stevia

1 teaspoon cinnamon

Instructions:

1. Preheat oven to 400°F.
2. Place parchment paper on a large cookie sheet.
3. Peel and slice sweet potatoes.
4. Toss with oil, stevia, and cinnamon until thoroughly coated.
5. Bake 20-30 minutes. Baking time will depend upon whether you like your chips soft or crispy.

Turnip Fries - V GF

These are so delicious you will not even miss having regular French fries. Added benefits of turnip fries over the traditional kind are that they are baked not fried and that the carb and calorie content are also much lower than that of a regular potato.

Ingredients:
4 medium turnips
2 tablespoons avocado oil
1 teaspoon chili powder
1 teaspoon paprika
½ teaspoon garlic powder
½ teaspoon sea salt
1/8 teaspoon cayenne pepper

Instructions:
1. Preheat oven to 425°F.
2. Line a large cookie sheet with parchment paper.
3. Peel your turnips and use a French fry cutter or sharp knife to cut turnips into French fry like pieces.
4. Put the turnips into a large mixing bowl and add seasoning.
5. Toss the turnips with the seasoning until well mixed.
6. Place on parchment paper.
7. Put fries into the oven for 15 minutes, flip them over, and bake for 15 more minutes or until golden brown and crispy.

No Better Chocolate Chip Cookies - P GF C

(Adapted from the Ambitious Kitchen)

Yields approximately 2 dozen cookies.

Ingredients:
1½ cups Namaste Gluten-Free Perfect Blend Flour
½ cup gluten-free oat flour
1 tsp baking soda
2/3 cup refined coconut oil
1¼ coconut palm sugar
1 organic omega-3 egg
1 organic omega-3 egg yolk
3 teaspoons pure vanilla
1 cup chocolate chips (I prefer dark chocolate.)

Instructions:
1. Preheat oven to 350°F.
2. Mix oat flour, baking soda, and salt together in one bowl.
3. Melt your coconut oil.
4. Mix melted coconut oil and coconut palm sugar together until creamy.
5. Blend in egg, egg yolk, and vanilla. Beat for 2-3 minutes with mixer, until no lumps appear.
6. Add flour mixture and blend until combined.
7. Toss in chocolate chips and fold into batter.
8. Place 1 inch balls onto cookie sheet 2 inches apart.
9. If you like soft chewy cookies, bake 8-11 minutes. If you like your cookies crispy, bake them 12-13 minutes or until golden brown.
10. Let your cookies cool for up to 5 minutes.

Nanna Cake - F C GF

Ingredients:

1½ cups coconut flour

1½ teaspoons aluminum-free baking powder

¾ teaspoon aluminum-free baking soda

1 teaspoon ground cinnamon

½ teaspoon fine sea salt

1 cup egg whites

⅔ cup coconut crystals

2 cups coconut milk

1 tablespoon apple cider vinegar

3 large very ripe bananas

¼ cup MCT oil or melted coconut oil

2 teaspoons pure vanilla

½ cup walnuts, chopped (optional)

Instructions:

1. Preheat oven to 375°F.
2. Lightly grease a 9x9 pan.
3. Put a tablespoon of apple cider vinegar into ½ cup of coconut milk and let it set until the milk begins to curdle. It will sort of have the consistency of buttermilk.
4. In a small bowl, beat eggs, vanilla, and bananas.
5. Pour in melted coconut oil and buttermilk-like mixture.
6. In a large bowl, mix together the flour, baking powder, baking soda, and cinnamon.
7. Add buttermilk-like mixture to the flour mixture in large bowl and beat until smooth.
8. Add in walnuts.
9. Pour batter into the pan and smooth out with spatula until even.
10. Bake for 18-22 minutes or until a toothpick comes out clean.
11. Cool cake in the pan 10 minutes. Remove from pan. Cool completely on wire rack and cut into 16 squares.

Hot Cinnamon Apple Crisp - P F C GF

This will make your kitchen smell great!

Ingredients:
5 large baking apples
¼ cup avocado, coconut, or pure olive oil
1 tablespoon lemon juice
2 teaspoons pumpkin pie spice
½ cup stevia
⅛ teaspoon sea salt
⅓ cup almond flour
1 scoop vanilla IsaLean
½ cup gluten-free rolled oats
½ teaspoon aluminum-free baking soda
½ teaspoon aluminum-free baking powder

Instructions:
1. Preheat oven to 350°F.
2. Peel and core baking apples. (My favorite kinds for this are Jonathan, Honeycrisp. or Granny Smith.)
3. Slice apples into thin slices. (This will make it easier for them to thoroughly bake and not be crunchy.)
4. In a large bowl, mix together sliced apples, lemon juice, and pumpkin pie spice until apples are well coated.
5. Lightly grease an 8x8 baking dish.
6. Bake the apple mixture without the crumb top for approximately 10 minutes.
7. Mix together all of the dry ingredients together with the oil of choice until crumbly.
8. Remove the apples from the oven. Sprinkle the dry crumbly mixture evenly over top of the apples.
9. Bake for 20-25 more minutes or until golden brown.

Dark Chocolate Protein Pudding - P C GF

Ingredients:

3 large ripe avocados

½ cup coconut or almond milk (unsweetened)

½ cup stevia

¼ cup coconut palm sugar

2 scoops vanilla IsaPro

1 teaspoon pure vanilla

1/3 cup Hershey's dark chocolate cocoa powder

Instructions:

1. Slice 3 large ripe avocados in half and pop out the seeds.
2. Scoop out the inside of the avocado and place into Ninja 1000 or a food processor.
3. Measure out the rest of the ingredients and put them in Ninja 1000 or a food processor.
4. Blend until smooth and creamy.

Slimming Lemonade - F

Yields 1 serving.

Ingredients:
1 lemon
8 ounces water
2-3 drops of liquid stevia
Crushed ice

Instructions:
1. Squeeze the juice of one lemon into water.
2. Add stevia and ice.

Linda's Banana-berry Workout Muffins - P F C

Pre or Post Workout Meal

Yields 12 Muffins.

Ingredients:
3 large ripe bananas
4 egg whites
2 tablespoons applesauce (unsweetened)
1/3 cup almond milk (unsweetened)
½ cup xylitol
1 teaspoon vanilla
½ teaspoon cinnamon
1 teaspoon sea salt
½ teaspoon baking soda
1 teaspoon aluminum-free baking powder
2 scoops vanilla IsaLean protein powder
2 cups gluten-free oat flour (or blend your own oat flour, processed to fine crumbs in blender)
1 cup frozen blueberries

Instructions:
1. Preheat oven to 350°F.
2. Mash bananas in a large mixing bowl with a fork.
3. Add egg whites, milk, sugar, salt, cinnamon, vanilla, baking soda, and aluminum-free baking powder to the bananas.
4. Beat well with whisk.
5. Gently blend the protein, flour, and oats into the banana mixture and stir for 20 seconds or until moistened.
6. Pour batter into lined or greased muffin pan, about ½ inch from the top.
7. Bake for 25 minutes or until a toothpick inserted near the middle of the center muffin comes out clean.
8. Let cool for 5 minutes before removing from pan.

Waffles - P C GF

Ingredients:

1½ cups almond flour

1 tablespoon arrowroot powder

½ teaspoon aluminum-free baking soda

¼ teaspoon sea salt

6 tablespoons egg whites

¼ cup coconut milk (unsweetened)

1 tablespoon coconut palm sugar

Instructions:

1. Preheat a waffle iron to medium.
2. In a large bowl, mix together the almond flour, arrowroot, baking soda, and salt.
3. In a small bowl, beat eggs, milk, and stevia until batter is smooth and creamy.
4. Grease and preheat your waffle iron. Fill preheated waffle iron with about ⅓ cup batter. Serve immediately with blueberry syrup.

Protein Pancakes - P C

Ingredients:

2 scoops vanilla IsaPro

3 egg whites

¼ cup gluten-free oatmeal, uncooked

¼ cup coconut milk (unsweetened)

Instructions:

1. Beat all ingredients together in a mixing bowl until smooth.
2. Pour mixture into a greased (with good fat) and heated skillet.
3. Cook on medium-low until the pancake begins to bubble on top. Flip.
4. Cook until golden brown.

Blueberry Syrup - F

Ingredients:

2 cups blueberries

½ cup water

2 tablespoons lemon juice

Instructions:

1. Cook on medium-low heat until blueberries begin to bubble.
2. Turn down to low and simmer until blueberries become syrup-like.
3. Sweeten to taste with stevia.

Dark Chocoholic Protein Bars - P C F

Ingredients:

1 cup Namaste Gluten-Free Perfect Blend Flour

¾ cup organic egg whites

2 scoops chocolate Isagenix IsaPro protein powder

½ cup stevia

½ teaspoon aluminum-free baking soda

¼ teaspoon sea salt

1 cup organic applesauce (unsweetened)

3 tablespoons Hershey's dark chocolate cocoa (unsweetened)

½ cup coconut milk (unsweetened)

Instructions:

1. Preheat oven to 350°F.
2. Mix dry ingredients together in a large bowl.
3. Mix wet ingredients together in a medium sized bowl.
4. Mix wet and dry ingredients together until smooth and creamy.
5. Spray 8x8 baking dish with a nonstick butter spray.
6. Pour batter into dish and spread evenly.
7. Bake 20-30 minutes in oven or until toothpick comes out clean.
8. Cut into 20 squares and serve once completely cooled.

Fudge Topping

Instructions:

1. Mix together 1 tablespoon of unsweetened cocoa mixture with 2 tablespoons of coconut milk and some stevia to sweeten.
2. Heat the fudge topping for 10-20 seconds in microwave.
3. Drizzle fudge sauce over the strawberries and chocolate protein bar.

Banana Walnut Protein Bars - P C F GF

Ingredients:

1 cup Namaste Gluten-Free Perfect Blend Flour

2 scoops vanilla Isagenix IsaPro protein powder

¼ teaspoon sea salt

½ teaspoon aluminum-free baking soda

2 large ripe bananas, mashed

¾ cup organic egg whites

½ cup stevia

1 cup organic applesauce (unsweetened)

½ cup coconut milk (unsweetened)

½ cup walnut pieces

Instructions:

1. Preheat oven to 350°F.
2. Mix dry ingredients in large bowl.
3. Mash 2 ripe bananas with a fork.
4. Mix liquid ingredients and bananas together in a small bowl.
5. Add wet ingredients to dry ingredients and mix together.
6. Mix wet and dry ingredients until smooth and creamy.
7. Spray 8x8 baking dish with nonstick butter spray.
8. Pour batter into dish and spread evenly. Pour ingredients into dish.
9. Bake 25-20 minutes or until toothpick comes out clean.
10. Cut into 16 squares and serve once completely cooled.

Pumpkin Apple Streusel Protein Bars - P F C

Ingredients:

2 cups Namaste Gluten-Free Perfect Blend Flour

2 scoops vanilla Isagenix IsaPro protein powder

½ cup stevia

2 teaspoons pumpkin pie spice

1 teaspoon aluminum-free baking powder

1 teaspoon aluminum-free baking soda

½ teaspoon sea salt

1 teaspoon pure vanilla

¾ cup organic egg whites

1 15-ounce can of pumpkin

½ cup coconut milk (unsweetened)

1 cup organic applesauce (unsweetened)

1 cup apples, chopped

1 cop nuts, chopped (optional)

Streusel Topping:

½ cup Namaste flour

¼ cup olive oil

½ cup gluten-free oats

½ cup stevia

¾ cup gluten-free quick oats

¾ teaspoon aluminum-free baking soda

½ teaspoon aluminum-free baking powder

Instructions:

1. Preheat oven to 350°F.
2. Mix all dry ingredients in large bowl.
3. Mix wet ingredients in a smaller bowl.
4. Add wet ingredients to dry ingredients and mix together.
5. Spray 13x9 baking dish with nonstick olive oil spray.
6. Pour batter into dish and spread evenly.
7. Mix all streusel topping ingredients together with a fork until crumbly.
8. Sprinkle evenly on top.

9.   Bake 30-35 minutes or until toothpick comes out clean and streusel top is golden brown.

10. Cut into 20 squares and serve once completely cooled

Butternutter Protein Bars - P F C

Ingredients:

½ cup stevia

2 teaspoons pumpkin pie spice

1 teaspoon aluminum-free baking powder

1 teaspoon aluminum-free baking soda

½ teaspoon sea salt

1 teaspoon pure vanilla

1 cup organic applesauce (unsweetened)

¾ cup organic egg whites

2 cups butternut squash

2 cups gluten-free oat flour (or blend your own oat flour, processed to fine crumbs in blender)

2 scoops vanilla Isagenix IsaPro protein powder

½ cup coconut milk (unsweetened)

½ cup chopped nuts, apples, or dark chocolate chips (optional)

Instructions:

1. Preheat oven to 350°F.
2. Mix dry ingredients in large bowl.
3. Mix wet ingredients in a smaller bowl.
4. Add wet ingredients to dry ingredients and mix together.
5. Spray 13X9 baking dish with nonstick butter spray.
6. Pour ingredients into dish.
7. Bake 30-35 minutes or until toothpick comes out clean.
8. Cut into 20 squares and serve once completely cooled.

Peanut Butter Protein Bars - P C F GF

Ingredients:

⅓ cup PB2 powder

1 cup Namaste Gluten-Free Perfect Blend Flour

2 scoops vanilla IsaPro protein powder

¼ teaspoon sea salt

½ teaspoon aluminum-free baking soda

¾ cup organic egg whites

½ cup stevia

1 cup organic applesauce (unsweetened)

½ cup coconut milk (unsweetened)

Instructions:

1. Preheat oven to 350°F.
2. Mix dry ingredients in large bowl.
3. Mix wet ingredients in a smaller bowl.
4. Add wet ingredients to dry ingredients and mix together until smooth and creamy.
5. Spray 8x8 baking dish with nonstick butter spray.
6. Pour batter into dish and spread evenly. Pour ingredients into dish.
7. Bake 25-20 minutes or until toothpick comes out clean.
8. Cut into 16 squares and serve once completely cooled

Peanut Butter Chocolate Protein Bars - P C F GF

Ingredients:

½ cup PB2 Powder

3 tablespoons Hershey's dark cocoa powder

2 cups Namaste Gluten-Free Perfect Blend Flour

2 scoops vanilla IsaPro protein powder

¼ teaspoon sea salt

½ teaspoon aluminum-free baking soda

¾ cup organic egg whites

½ cup stevia

1 cup organic applesauce (unsweetened)

½ cup coconut milk (unsweetened)

Instructions:

1. Preheat oven to 350°F.
2. Mix dry ingredients in large bowl.
3. Mix liquid ingredients in a smaller bowl.
4. Add wet ingredients to dry ingredients and mix together until smooth and creamy.
5. Spray 13x9 baking dish with nonstick butter spray.
6. Pour batter into two separate mixing bowls.
7. Mix PB2 powder in one bowl and Hershey's dark chocolate cocoa in the other.
8. Pour peanut butter batter on the bottom layer and spread evenly in 13x9 pan.
9. Pour Hershey's dark cocoa batter on the top layer and spread evenly over peanut butter.
10. Bake 30-35 minutes or until toothpick comes out clean.
11. Cut into 20 squares and serve once completely cooled.

Lemonade Protein Bar - P F C

Ingredients:

1 cup Namaste Gluten-Free Perfect Blend Flour

2 scoops vanilla IsaPro protein powder

¼ teaspoon sea salt

½ teaspoon aluminum-free baking soda

½ cup lemon juice

1 teaspoon lemon zest

4 packets True Lemon

¾ cup organic egg whites

½ cup stevia

1 cup organic applesauce (unsweetened)

Instructions:

1. Preheat oven to 350°F.
2. Mix dry ingredients in large bowl.
3. Mix wet ingredients in a smaller bowl.
4. Mix wet and dry ingredients together until smooth and creamy.
5. Spray 8x8 baking dish with nonstick butter spray.
6. Pour batter into dish and spread evenly.
7. Bake 25-20 minutes or until toothpick comes out clean.
8. Cut into 16 squares and serve once completely cooled.

Healthy Holiday Recipes

Pumpkin Spice Cookies – P C F

This recipe is so simple and delicious you won't even feel like you're missing out at the holidays.

Ingredients:

1 cup canned or fresh pumpkin or 1 cup sweet potato, mashed

1 packet or ½ cup vanilla IsaPro

½ cup Namaste Flour Gluten-Free Perfect Flour Blend

1 teaspoon aluminum-free baking soda

1 teaspoon ground cinnamon

½ teaspoon ground nutmeg

¼ teaspoon ground cloves

2 cups gluten-free quick oats

½ cup organic applesauce (unsweetened)

½ cup stevia

1 large organic omega-3 egg

1 teaspoon pure vanilla

Optional - chopped walnuts, raisins, dark chocolate chips

Instructions:

1. Preheat oven to 350°F.
2. Mix all of the wet ingredients together in a small bowl.
3. Mix all of the dry ingredients together in a large mixing bowl.
4. Combine the wet and dry ingredients together until mixed well.
5. Drop the dough by spoonful onto a parchment paper lined cookie sheet. Bake for 10-12 minutes or until golden brown.
6. Remove cookies from the oven and let them cool before putting them on a plate.

Optional - add in walnuts, raisins, cacao nibs, or dark chocolate chips.

Pumpkin Spice Latte – C P

You no longer have to stand at the coffee window and drool. Now, you can make your own healthy pumpkin spice latte!

Ingredients:

2 cups coconut milk (unsweetened)

2 cups black organic coffee or 2 shots espresso

Stevia or coconut palm sugar (sweeten to your taste)

1 teaspoon cinnamon

½ teaspoon ginger

¼ teaspoon cloves

¼ teaspoon nutmeg

1½ teaspoon pure vanilla

½ cup cooked pumpkin

Instructions:

1. In a medium saucepan on medium-low heat, mix together the spices, pumpkin, and coconut milk.
2. Stir to keep it from sticking until pumpkin milk is steamy.
3. I like to send my hot milk mixture through the blender to make it nice and frothy.
4. Pour your hot coffee into your pumpkin spice mixture.
5. Stir and serve.

Gluten-Free, Dairy-Free Pie Crust - C GF

Crust Ingredients:

1 cup Namaste Gluten-Free Perfect Blend Flour

¼ teaspoon sea salt

¼ teaspoon aluminum-free baking soda

¼ cup avocado oil

2 tablespoons honey

1 teaspoon pure vanilla

Instructions:

1. Preheat Oven to 325°F.
2. Mix together dry ingredients in a small bowl. Then mix in wet ingredients until combined well.
3. Press into 9-inch pie pan.
4. Bake 10 minutes or until golden brown at 325°F.

Coconut Flour Pie Crust - P C GF

Ingredients:

¼ cup cold organic grass-fed butter

2 tablespoons refined coconut oil, solid

½ cup coconut flour

1 tablespoon water

Pinch of sea salt

1 organic egg white, beaten

Instructions:

1. Preheat oven to 325°F.
2. In a medium sized bowl, cut the butter and coconut oil with a fork until mixed well.
3. Mix all of the other ingredients together except egg whites.
4. Mix the dough together with your hands and press into 9-inch pie plate.
5. When you are done, beat the egg white until frothy.
6. Brush the pie crust with egg white just before filling.
7. 10 minutes or until golden brown at 325°F.

Honey Almond Crust - P C GF

(Inspired by Charles Poliquin)

Ingredients:

1½ cups almond flour

¼ teaspoon sea salt

¼ teaspoon baking soda

¼ cup avocado oil

1 tablespoon honey

1 omega-3 egg

1 teaspoon vanilla

Instructions:

1. Preheat oven to 325°F.
2. Mix together dry ingredients. Then mix in wet ingredients until combined well.
3. Press into 9-inch pie pan.
4. Bake 10 minutes or until golden brown at 325°F.

Peanut Butter Crème Pie - P C GF

Filling Ingredients:

½ cup PB2 Powder

Crunchy peanut butter (without any added salt or sugar)

Crushed peanuts (optional)

1 cup coconut palm sugar

¼ Namaste Gluten-Free Perfect Blend Flour

3 omega-3 egg yolks

1/8 teaspoon sea salt

2 cups coconut milk

1 teaspoon vanilla

Pie crust of choice

Instructions:

1. Mix all ingredients together with a wire whisk until well blended.
2. Cook on medium heat 10 minutes or until it begins to thicken.
3. Stir continually to keep from sticking.
4. Spread some natural peanut butter on the crust or swirl through the peanut butter crème filling.
5. Pour into baked pie shell.
6. Sprinkle some crushed peanuts on top (optional).
7. Cool in fridge.

Chocolate Crème Pie - P C GF

Filling Ingredients:

½ cup Hershey's special dark cocoa

1 cup coconut palm sugar

¼ Namaste Gluten-Free Perfect Blend Flour

3 omega-3 egg yolks

1/8 teaspoon sea salt

2 cups coconut milk

1 teaspoon vanilla

Pie crust of choice

Instructions:

1. Mix all ingredients together with a wire whisk until well blended.
2. Cook on medium heat 10 minutes or until it begins to thicken.
3. Stir continually to keep from sticking.
4. Pour into baked pie shell.
5. Cool in fridge.

Pumpkin Crème Filling - P C GF

Filling Ingredients:

½ cup pumpkin

1 cup coconut palm sugar

¼ cup coconut flour

3 organic omega-3 egg yolks

1/8 teaspoon sea salt

2 cups coconut milk

1 teaspoon pure vanilla

Pie crust of choice

Instructions:

1. Mix all ingredients together with a wire whisk until well blended.
2. Cook on medium heat 10 minutes or until it begins to thicken.
3. Stir continually to keep from sticking.
4. Pour into baked pie shell.
5. Cool in fridge

Banana Coconut Crème Filling - P C GF

Filling Ingredients:

3 large ripe bananas, sliced

2 scoops vanilla IsaLean protein powder

1 cup coconut palm sugar

¼ cup coconut flour

3 organic omega-3 egg yolks

1/8 teaspoon sea salt

2 cups coconut milk

2 teaspoons pure vanilla

Pie crust of choice

Instructions:

1. Mix all ingredients together with a wire whisk until well blended.
2. Cook on medium heat 10 minutes or until it begins to thicken.
3. Stir continually to keep from sticking.
4. Slice bananas and place evenly in pie shell.
5. Pour mixture into baked pie shell.
6. Cool in fridge.

Sweet Potato Pie Filling - P C GF

Filling Ingredients:

1½ pounds sweet potatoes

½ cup coconut palm sugar

1½ teaspoons cinnamon

1/8 teaspoon ground ginger

1/8 teaspoon ground nutmeg

Pinch of ground cloves

½ cup evaporated coconut milk (unsweetened)

½ tablespoon pure vanilla

1 egg

2 egg whites

Gluten-free pie crust

Instructions:

1. Peel and chop your sweet potatoes into chunks.
2. Boil sweet potatoes for 20 minutes or so, until tender.
3. Mash and mix them together with butter and spices.
4. Beat egg whites into sweet potato mixture until smooth and creamy.
5. Pour into baked gluten-free pie crust and bake at 425°F for 15 minutes. Turn down heat and bake at 350°F for 30-35 more minutes or until toothpick comes out clean.

Pumpkin Pie (Gluten-Free, Sugar-Free) - P C

Filling Ingredients:

15 ounces pumpkin

1 teaspoon cinnamon

½ teaspoon ground ginger

½ teaspoon nutmeg

½ teaspoon sea salt

1 14-ounce can of evaporated coconut milk

1 cup coconut crystals

Pie crust of choice

Instructions:

1. Preheat oven to 425°F. Prepare pie crust.
2. Place pumpkin and spices into small saucepan on medium-low and stir constantly.
3. Heat filling until it begins to bubble.
4. Place eggs and milk into pumpkin spice mixture.
5. Whisk mixture until thoroughly combined and pour into unbaked pie shell.
6. Bake 13 minutes at 425°F. Reduce temperature to 350°F and bake 30 more minutes or until knife comes out clean. (Cover edges of pie crust with aluminum foil so edges don't get overly brown.)

Oatmeal Raisin Cookies - P F C GF

Ingredients:

1/3 cup gluten-free oats

1 scoop vanilla IsaLean pro

1 egg white

¼ cup applesauce (unsweetened)

¼ teaspoon baking powder

¼ teaspoon cinnamon

¼ cup stevia

Chopped apple, walnuts, or raisins (optional)

Instructions:

1. Preheat oven to 350°F.
2. Grease baking pan.
3. In a bowl, mix all ingredients together.
4. You may need to add a touch of water to make the mixture into a batter.
5. Drop by spoonful onto baking sheet.
6. Bake for 10-15 minutes or until lightly browned.

12
Healthy Body, Healthy Skin

SOS Beauty Boot Camp

I have provided some great organic beauty recipes for you where you can grab the ingredients right out of your pantry. Make fresh, healthy, all natural, and inexpensive beauty products in the privacy of your own home. Eating healthier and using products without synthetics, parabens, chemicals, and a whole host of preservatives will truly create beauty from the inside out. When you live a life that brings you joy and health, it almost certainly brings beauty to the forefront.

"There is no cosmetic for beauty like happiness."
-Maria Mitchell

Vanilla Coconut Cleanser

Ingredients:

3 teaspoons coconut oil

5 drops vanilla oil

1 teaspoon olive oil

1 teaspoon glycerin

2 teaspoons water

Instructions:

1. Melt ingredients together on a low heat.
2. Once melted, remove from heat, add in vanilla oil, and beat with a whisk for five minutes.
3. Transfer to airtight jar when cooled.

Lemon Astringent

Ingredients:

4 teaspoons lemon juice

8 teaspoons witch hazel

½ teaspoon peppermint extract

2 teaspoons rubbing alcohol

Tingly Toner

Ingredients:

1 cup purified water

4 tablespoons apple cider vinegar

10 drops essential mint oil

Instructions:

Mix all of the ingredients together. This toner will leave your skin feeling clean, tight, and refreshed. Place in an airtight jar.

Bedtime Facial Scrub:

Ingredients:

1 cup organic cane sugar

½ cup jojoba oil

1 teaspoon vitamin E oil

½ teaspoon pure vanilla

15 drops lavender essential oil

Instructions:

Mix all the ingredients well. Keep facial sugar scrub in an airtight jar.

Nature's Mask

Ingredients:

1 tablespoon (approximate) bentonite clay

1-2 tablespoons (or more) Bragg's apple cider vinegar

Instructions:

Mix clay and ACV together until it forms a paste. If it is too thick, add a little bit more ACV or water. Spread it on your face staying away from your eyes until you have a thin layer completely covering the skin. Leave on for 15-20 minutes or until you feel your face tighten and the mask begins to crack. For extra facelift benefits, try not to smile until the mask has worked its magic. Your skin will feel baby smooth.

Egg On Your Face

Ingredients:

2 tablespoons baking soda

1 egg white

Instructions:

Mix baking soda and egg white together until smooth and pasty. Apply directly to your face and leave for 20 minutes. Be careful not to ingest the egg whites as sometimes you can get salmonella from raw eggs.

Lemon-Lime Sugar Scrub

This recipe is both cleansing and detoxifying. Lemon is very detoxifying to the body and will also help brighten the skin. This will help you slough off and shed dead and dry skin cells, leaving the body feeling invigorated and naturally moisturized. It's best to do this where you can rinse off the sugar and not worry about getting it everywhere.

Ingredients:

2 teaspoons rubbing alcohol
6 drops of lemon oil
6 drops of lime oil
½-1 cup organic cane sugar
1 cup grape seed, olive, jojoba, apricot, or almond oil

Instructions:

Mix all the ingredients well. Keep lemon scrub in an airtight jar.

Salt Scrub

Ingredients:

20-30 drops essential oil of choice
4 cups grape seed, olive, jojoba, apricot, or almond oil
20-30 drops essential oil of choice

Instructions:

Mix all the ingredients well. Keep salt scrub in an airtight jar.

Salt of the Earth (Detox Bath)

Ingredients:

½ cup Celtic salt

½ cup Epsom salt

½ cup aluminum-free baking soda

½ cup Bragg's apple cider vinegar

5 drops eucalyptus oil

5 drop juniper oil

Instructions:

Mix together all of your ingredients and put into a pitcher. Fill tub with warm/hot water and pour into water. Epsom salts are great for removing toxins and restoring magnesium levels in the body. Soak for approximately 10-20 minutes or as desired.

Oxygen Bath

Ingredients:

1 cup Epsom salts

½-1 cup 35% hydrogen peroxide

10 drops of your favorite essential oil

Instructions:

Start with a small amount of hydrogen peroxide. You don't want to use too much if you're not used to this type of bath. You might not want to do this at night; this type of soak is very stimulating and oxygenating to the body so it could potentially keep you awake. Start with a 10 minute soak. As you get used to taking this sort of bath, you may eventually work your way up to 20 or 30 minutes.

13
Work it Out

SOS S.W.E.A.T. Selections

Exercise Descriptions - You can find all exercises in the glossary. Check out Linda Mitchell's CHICKFIT Channel on Vimeo or YouTube for the free #SOS S.W.E.A.T. exercise video glossary. You will find definitions for all the exercises and/or videos. The videos are constantly being updated as new workouts are provided. If you can't find them in the glossary or videos, try your computer's search engine. I try to stay consistent with the names of exercises so they are universal. You can also Google the exercises as I used common universal terms and names for all of the exercise selections.

Doing full body workouts such as our SOS functional training will fire up more muscle groups at a time, ultimately burning more calories per workout session. When you decrease the total volume per muscle group, you will automatically increase the recovery rate. We will accelerate the calories burned because we are able to work out metabolically more often. We will be training like an athlete trains, using their full body as a unit rather than lifting a five pound dumbbell. We will be using your body weight to train which will give you quick results. There are 21 high octane workouts in the SOS S.W.E.A.T. Selections. Please make sure to warm-up for ten minutes prior to all workouts to get the blood flowing gradually, to increase range of motion, limber up, and prevent injury. You can use the dynamic warm-up provided on page 204.

Equipment Needed:

TRX Suspension Trainer (www.trxtraining.com)
Kettlebells (www.onnit.com/fitness)
Dumbbells, Plyo Box, Medicine Ball (http://www.ragefitness.com)
Jump Rope, Weight Plates (www.roguefitness.com)
TKO Cardio Pump Set (https://www.tko.com/products/tko-cardio-pump-set)

Dynamic Warm-Up

High Knees down and Back Pedal back, x 3 sets
Butt Kickers down and Back Pedal back, x 3 sets
Frankensteins down and back
Inch Worms, 10 reps
Pogos, 10 reps
Hip Circles
Knee Hugs
Walking Quad Stretch
Leg Swings

High Octane

Run down, Back Pedal x 3 sets, Jump Squat at each end 10 (Total 60 Burpees)
Skip across, Back Pedal x 3 sets, TRX 1 Leg Jammers 30 at 1 end (Total 90, 1 Leg Jammers)
Skip for height, Back Pedal x 3 sets, 10 Push-Ups at each end (Total 60 Push-Ups)
Skip with Twist, Back Pedal x 3 sets, 10 V-Ups at each end (Total 60 V-Ups)
Karaoke down and back, 20 Mountain Climbers at each end, x 3 sets (Total 60 Mountain Climbers)
Shuffle down and back, Burpees 10 at each end, x 3 sets (Total 60 Burpees)
Long Jump down and back
Frog Hop down and back
Lunges down and back
Bear Crawl down and back

Sneaky 6

Equipment:
Dumbbells

Plyo Box

Shuffle Add On

Shuffle down, 6 Jump Lunges ES (Each Side), Shuffle back

Shuffle down, 6 Jump Lunges ES, 6 Burpees Shuffle back

Shuffle down, 6 Jump Lunges ES, 6 Burpees, 6 Frog Jumps, Shuffle back

Shuffle down, 6 Jump Lunges ES, 6 Burpees, 6 Frog Jumps, 6 Tuck Jumps, Shuffle back

Shuffle down, 6 Jump Lunges ES, 6 Burpees, 6 Frog Jumps, 6 Tuck Jumps, 6 Box Jumps, Shuffle back

Shuffle down, 6 Jump Lunges ES, 6 Burpees, 6 Frog Jumps, 6 Tuck Jumps, 6 Box Jumps, 6 Split Laps, Shuffle back

Shuffle down, 6 Jump Lunges ES, 6 Burpees, 6 Frog Jumps, 6 Tuck Jumps, 6 Box Jumps, 6 Backwards Frog Hops, Shuffle Back

Use dumbbells but keep in mind you will be doing 30 reps so use ¾ of the weight you're used to using for 15 reps. Example: Shoulder Press 20 lbs. regular 15 reps, 15 lbs. higher reps 30

Shoulder Press, 30 reps

Squats, 30 reps

1 Leg Split Squat, 30 reps

Push-Ups, 30 reps

Bent Knee Sit-Ups, 30 reps

Lateral Raise, 30 reps

V-Ups, 30 reps

Pec Fly, 30 reps

Tricep Dips, 30 reps

Bent Over Row, 30 reps

Upright Row, 30 reps

Lucky 7

Equipment:
TRX Suspension Trainer,
Plyo Box

Round 1
1 minute work - 20 second rest
TRX Squat Jumps
TRX Wall Sits
TRX Front Squats

Round 2
TRX Hamstring Curls
TRX Pistol Squats ES
Box Jumps

Round 3
TRX Curtsy Lunge ES
Ninja Burpees
TRX Rear Fly

Round 4
TRX Pike-Ups
TRX Suspension Jammers ES
Bear Crawl

Round 5
TRX Calf Raises
Russian Twists
TRX Pull-Ups

Round 6
Sprinters Start ES
TRX Row to Bicep Curl
TRX Triceps Press

Round 7
TRX Swimmers Pull
TRX Plank
Sit-Ups

8 Minute Metabolic Circuit

(For results, don't go easy here!)
Jump Lunges, 1 minute
Burpees, 20 reps
Mountain Climbers, 1 minute
Skaters, 1 minute
Groiners, 30 seconds
Straight Leg Lifts, 20 reps
Walking Lunges, 20 sets (ES)
Jumping Jack Squat, 20 reps
Russian Twist, 20 sets (ES)
Crunches, 20 reps
If you have a tight schedule this is a great way to get a metabolic workout in
a short amount of time. One time through is a great 8 minute workout.
Repeat three times for a 24 minute workout.

SOS Beast/Mode-Functional
Box Jumps for Breakfast

Equipment:
Plyo Box

1 Shuffle down and back, 8 Jump Lunges ESEE (Each Side & Each End)
8 Box Jumps
30 Tuck Jumps
8 Box Jumps
30 Mountain Climbers
8 Box Jumps
15 Plyo Push-Ups

8 Box Jumps

Sprint 100 yards, x2

2 Shuffle down and back, 8 Tuck Jumps ESEE

8 Box Jumps

30 Tuck Jumps

8 Box Jumps

30 Mountain Climbers

8 Box Jumps

15 Plyo Push-Ups

Sprint 100 yards, x2

3 Shuffle down and back, 8 Burpees ESEE

8 Box Jumps

30 Tuck Jumps

8 Box Jumps

30 Mountain Climbers

8 Box Jumps

Sprint 100 yards, x2

15 Plyo Push-Ups

4 Shuffle down and back, 8 V-Ups ESEE

8 Box Jumps

30 Tuck Jumps

8 Box Jumps

30 Mountain Climbers

8 Box Jumps

15 Plyo Push-Ups

Sprint 100 yards, x2

SOS Beast/Mode-Functional

Luscious Legs

Equipment:

Dumbbells

Medicine Ball

Weighted Walking Lunge D&B (down and back)
Bear Crawl D&B
Weighted Burpees, 15 Reps
Walking 1 Leg Lunge Right D&B
Walking 1 Leg Lunge Left D&B
Bear Crawl D&B
Weighted Burpees, 15 Reps
Weighted Step-Up Right, 15 Reps
Weighted Step-Up Left, 15 Reps
Bear Crawl D&B
Weighted Burpees, 15 Reps
Weighted Reverse Lunge Right, 15 Reps
Weighted Reverse Lunge Left, 15 Reps
Bear Crawl D&B
Weighted Burpees, 15 Reps
Weighted Side Lunge ES, 15 Reps
Bear Crawl D&B
Weighted Burpees, 15 Reps
Repeat 2x

AB Segment

Reverse Curls with MB (Medicine Ball)
Oblique Heel Touch
Opposite Hand to Leg Touch (Half V-Ups)
20 each, x3 sets

Perfect Ten Workout

Equipment:
Medicine Ball
Dumbbells
Battle Jump Rope
TRX Suspension Trainer

The Perfect Ten Workout is 10 exercises, done in 10 reps each, for 10 rounds.
Slam Ball Slams
TRX 1 Leg Jammer
Dumbbell Squat Jump
Burpee Plank Jack
Tuck Jumps
Mount Everest Climbers
Slam Ball Wall Ball Squat 'n' Throw
Battle Jump Rope, 100 skips
TRX Push-Up
Slam Ball Sit-Up

S.W.E.A.T. - Sister

Your partner picks the moves. Set the timer for 60 seconds. Rest for 20 seconds. Then you pick the moves, set the timer for 60 seconds, and then rest for 20 seconds.

Equipment:
Timer
Medicine Ball
Kettle Bell
TRX Suspension Trainer

Exercises:
Burpee Plank Jack
Kettlebell Snatch
Box Jumps
Triangle Hops
Bear Crawl
Sit-Ups
Kettlebell Swing
Inch Worms
Plank Walk

Medicine Ball Thrusters
Plank Shoulder Taps
Plank
Straight Leg V-Ups
Mountain Climbers
Tricep Dips
Decline Push-Ups
Bulgarian Lunge Hops
Turkish Get-Up
TRX Pull-Ups

100 Ways to Get Ridiculous

Equipment:
TRX Suspension Trainer

100 Jumping Jacks
100 Burpees
100 TRX Pull-Ups
100 Crunches
100 TRX Bicep Curls
100 Push-Ups
100 TRX Tricep Extensions
100 Russian Twists
100 Jumping Jack Squat Jumps
100 Alternating Side Kicks
100 Squat Thrusts
100 Jump Lunges
100 Sit-Ups
200 Crunches

Insane Chicks Workout!

Ding, Ding, Ding!
Insane Results

Equipment:
TRX Suspension Trainer
Dumbbells
TKO Cardio Pump Set

Jump Rope 2 minutes

Round 1
100 TKO Squats
10 V-Ups
15 TRX Jump Squats
30 second TRX Wall Sits
TRX Front Squats
Hand Release Push-Ups AMRAP (As Many Reps As Possible)

Round 2
75 TKO Squats
20 V-Ups
15 TRX Hamstring Curls
30 TRX Calf Raises
8 TRX Pistol Squats per leg
8 Man Makers with dumbbells

Round 3
50 TKO Squats
30 V-Ups
15 TRX Curtsy Lunges (Each Leg)
15 TRX Sprinter Starts (Each Leg)
Mountain Climber Crossovers

Round 4
25 TKO Squats
40 V-20 TRX Plank Pendulum Swings
20 TRX 1 Leg Jammers
Repeat for 3 rounds.
Ninja Burpees

Add-Ons

Equipment:

Plyo Box

Warm Up

Run down and back Pedal, 3x

Skip down and back Pedal, 3x

Carioca down and back, 20 Mountain Climbers ES, 3x

High Knees down, Butt Kickers back, 3x

Lunge down, Shuffle back, change sides 2x

Shuffle down, 5 Push-Ups, Shuffle back, 5 Push-Ups

Shuffle down, 5 Push-Ups, 5 X Jumps

Shuffle back, 5 Push-Ups, 5 X Jumps

Keep adding on until you complete the list 3 times through.

1. Push-Ups
2. X Jumps
3. Mountain Climbers
4. Skaters
5. Plank Jacks
6. Burpees
7. Plank Shoulder Taps
8. Jumping Jack Squats
9. Squat Thrusts
10. Box Jumps

Take It Outside

Run stadium steps, every one

Run stadium steps, every other one

Run stadium steps sideways, right side

Run stadium steps sideways, left side

Run stadium steps, every one

Skip stadium steps, every other one

Run stadium steps sideways, every other one, right side

Run stadium steps sideways, every other one, left side
Jump up steps
Run stadium steps, every one
Skip stadium steps, every other one
Skip stadium steps sideways, every other one, right side
Skip stadium steps sideways, every other one, left side
Repeat.

Burn, Baby, Burn

Sprint 100 yards 12x, 10 Push-Ups at each end
Sprint 75 yards 12x, 10 Sit-Ups at each end
Sprint 50 yards 12x, 10 Burpees at each end
Lunge 50 yards, Run 50 yards, 6x (length of a football field)

Burpee Add-Ons

Run down and back, 1 Burpee at each end
Run down and back, 2 Burpees at each end
Run down and back, 3 Burpees at each end
Run down and back, 4 Burpees at each end
Run down and back, 5 Burpees at each end
Run down and back, 6 Burpees at each end
Run down and back, 7 Burpees at each end
Run down and back, 8 Burpees at each end
Run down and back, 9 Burpees at each end
Run down and back, 10 Burpees at each end
Run down and back, 11 Burpees at each end
Run down and back, 12 Burpees at each end

Spell Your Whole Name

Equipment:
TRX Suspension Trainer
Medicine Ball
Plyo Box

A = 20 Medicine Ball Crunches

B = 15 Plyo Push-Ups

C = 50 Jumping Jacks

D = 2 minute Wall Sit

E = 30 TRX Squats

F = 15 Burpees

G = 20 Box Jumps

H = 20 Gorillas

I = 50 Plank Jacks

J = 15 V-Ups

K = 60 Mountain Climbers ES

L = 25 Burpees

M = 1 minute Wall Sit

N = 25 Burpees

O = Lateral Bear Crawl D&B

P = Triceps Pushups

Q = 30 Sit-Ups

R = 15 TRX Push-Ups (feet in Foot Cradles)

S = 30 Burpees

T = 50 Front Lunges ES

U = 30 Jump Lunges ES

V = 3 minute Wall Sit

W = 20 Burpees

X = 20 X Jumps

Y = 20 Triceps Dips

Z = 20 Step Ups ES

Full Body Meltdown

Equipment:

TRX Suspension Trainer

Battle Jump Rope

Kettlebells

Medicine Ball

1. Jump Rope, 2 minutes
   1 leg Stationary Jump Lunge, 30 sec ES
   Heavy Medicine Ball Slam, 2 minutes
   TRX Pull-Ups, 2 minutes
   Repeat.
2. Jump Rope, 2 minutes
   Kettlebell Swing, 2 minutes
   Heavy Medicine Ball Slam Side to Side, 2 minutes
   TRX Push-Ups, 2 minutes
   Repeat.
3. Jump Rope, 2 minutes
   Turkish Get Up with Kettlebell, 6 reps ES
   Heavy Medicine 1 Arm Push-Up (roll ball side to side), 2 minutes
   Repeat.
4. Jump Rope, 2 minutes
   20 V-Ups with Medicine Ball
   TRX Combo – Push-Up, Pec Fly, Roll Out, 2 minutes
   TRX Bicep Curls, 2 minutes

#SOS

Equipment:
TRX Suspension Trainer
Kettlebells
Dumbbells

Series 1
Sprint 60 sec
30 Burpees for time
15 Sit-Ups

Series 2
Sprint 60 sec
30 KB Swing

15 Push-Ups

Series 3

Run ½ mile

30 Burpees for time

30 Jump Lunges

Series 4

Sprint 60 sec

30 Mountain Climbers, ES

15 Push-Press

Series 5

Sprint 60 sec

30 Burpees for time

15 Frog Hops

Series 6

Run ½ mile

30 Burpees for time

15 TRX Pull-Up or Body Row

Fried in 30

Equipment:

Weight Plate

Run ½ mile

Walking Lunges, 3 minutes

Run ½ mile

Bear Crawl or Plate Push, 3 minutes

Run ½ mile

Burpees, 3 minutes

Run ½ mile

Push-Ups, 3 minutes

Run ½ mile

Plank, 3 minutes

The following cranks are short but intense body part focused workouts. These are designed to get you results in a short amount of time.

Arm Crank

3-5 rounds, 12 reps
Ninja Burpee
Hand Release Push-Ups
Shoulder Taps
Alternating Plank Walk
Tricep Dips

Leg Crank

3-5 rounds, 12 reps
Mt. Everest Climber
1 legged Burpee
Jump Lunge
X Jumps
Reverse Lunge

Ab Crank

Equipment:
Medicine Ball

3-5 rounds, 15 reps
Reverse Crunches with Medicine Ball
Oblique Heel Touchers
V-Ups
Suitcase
Russian Twists

WORDS TO MY S.W.E.A.T SISTERS

You've got to grab a hold of life with both hands because it is all over too soon. Life is short! Live, breath, and get your hands dirty!

You can't make everyone happy and you free yourself of a lot of stress, grief, and worry when you focus on what you can control, which is making yourself happy.

Staying vital is really all about pushing forward and setting goals regardless of the outcome. When you reach for something, you are one step closer to it and one step further away from where you used to be. Then, all of the sudden, you're on this journey and it's called amazing!

The heck with worrying about what other people think! Amaze yourself! Celebrate yourself each and every day by getting out there and living your life unabashedly and unapologetically by being your authentic self! Live loud!

WORKS CITED

Aller, G., Abete, Itziar., et al. "Starches, Sugars and Obesity." *PubMed Central*. US National Library of Medicine National Institutes of Health, 14 March 2011. Web.

Axe, Josh. "Eating Tilapia Is Worse than Eating Bacon." *DrAxe.com*. Dr. Axe. Web.

Bennett, Connie. "The Rats Who Preferred Sugar Over Cocaine." *HuffingtonPost.com*. HuffPost Healthy Living. The Huffington Post, 10 September 2014. Web.

Callahan, Christy. "Natural Calm Benefits." *livestrong.com*. Demand Media, 16 August 2013. Web.

Calorie Control Council. "Stuff the Bird, Not Yourself: How to Deal with the 3,000 Calorie Thanksgiving Meal." *CalorieControl.org*. Calorie Control Council. Web.

Coconut Research Center. "Coconut (Cocos Nucifera) The Tree of Life." *CoconutResearchCenter.com*. Coconut Research Center, 2004. Web.

"Did You Know That Raw Cacao Benefits Human Longevity and Health Without Negative Side Effects?" *Secrets-of-Longevity-in-Humans.com*. Secrets of Longevity, Govan Kilgour. Web.

Fife, Bruce. *The Coconut Oil Miracle*. Garden City: Avery Publishing, 2004. Print.

Gittleman, Ann Louise. "Why the Grapefruit Diet is Making a Comeback." *AnnLouise.com*. First Lady of Nutrition, Inc., 19 July 2012. Web.

"Glycemic Load Chart." *Natural Choices for You*. Natural Choices, Inc. Web.

Goldstein, Hesh. "MSG: Many Secrets Guarded (opinion)." *NaturalNews.com*. Natural News Network. Web.

Gunnar, Kris. "6 Proven Benefits of Apple Cider Vinegar (No. 3 is Best)." *AuthorityNutrition.com*. Authority   Nutrition, June 2014. Web.

Harvard University. "Glycemic Index and Glycemic Load for 100+ Foods." *Harvard Health Publications*. Harvard Medical School, 3 February 2015. Web.

Kadooka, Y., Sato, M. et al. "Regulation of Abdominal Adiposity by Probiotics (Lactobacillus Gasseri SBT2055) in Adults with Obese Tendencies in a Randomized Controlled Trial." *European Journal of Clinical Nutrition.* (2010): 64, 636-643. Print.

Lam, Michael. "Adrenal Fatigue Myths Part 1." *DrLam.com.* Adrenal Fatigue Center. Michael Lam, M.D. Web.

Lang, Susan S. "Eating Less Meat May Help Reduce Osteoporosis Risk, Studies Show." *News.Cornell.edu.* Cornell Chronicle. Cornell University, 14 November 1996. Web.

Maersk, Maria., Belza, Anita., et al. "Sucrose-Sweetened Beverages Increase Fat Storage in the Liver, Muscle, and Visceral Fat Depot: a 6-Mo Randomized Intervention Study." *ajcn.nutrition.org.* The American Journal of Clinical Nutrition. American Society for Nutrition, 1 November 2011. Web.

Manzella, Debra. "Glycemic Index Chart for Common Foods." *About.com.* 16 December 2014. Web.

Marković, Maria. "Creamy Chocolate Pie." *StrengthSensei.com.* Charles R. Poliquin, 16 June 2015. Web.

Mercola, Joseph M. "Artificial Sweeteners—More Dangerous Than You Ever Imagined." *Mercola.com.* Dr. Joseph Mercola, 13 October 2009. Web.

Mercola, Joseph M. "Coconut Oil Benefits: When Fat is Good For You." *HuffingtonPost.com.* The Huffington Post, 14 February 2011. Web.

Mercola, Joseph M. "News Flash: Acid Reflux Caused by Too Little Acid, Not Too Much." *Mercola.com.* Dr. Joseph Mercola, 25 April 2009.Web.

Mercola, Joseph M. "Probiotics Found to Help Your Gut's Immune System." *Mercola.com.* Dr. Joseph Mercola, 5 July 2008. Web.

Mercola, Joseph M. "Surprising Health Benefits of Vegetables." *Mercola.com.* Dr. Joseph Mercola, 8 September 2014. Web.

Mehmet, Oz. "Lose Belly Fat: Dr. Oz's 5 Tips for a Flatter Stomach." *HuffingtonPost.com.* The Huffington Post, 26 September 2014. Web.

Mimura, A., Suzuki, Y., Yazaki, S., et al. "Induction of Apoptosis in Human Leukemia Cells by Naturally Fermented Sugar Cane Vinegar (kibizu) of Amami Ohshima Island." *PubMed.gov.* US National Library of Medicine National Institutes of Health, 2004. Web.

Mitchell, Linda. "Isagenix Coffee." *lindalu7.isagenix.com.* Isagenix International, LLC. Web.

Nanda, K., Miyoshi, N., Nakamura, Y., et al. "Extract of Vinegar "Kurosu" from Unpolished Rice Inhibits the Proliferation of Human Cancer Cells." *PubMed.gov.* US National Library of Medicine National Institutes of Health, March 2004. Web.

Nettleton, JA., Lutsey, PL., Wang, Y., et al. "Diet Soda Intake and Risk of Incident Metabolic Syndrome and Type 2 Diabetes in the Multi-Ethnic Study of Atherosclerosis (MESA)." *PubMed.gov.* US National Library of Medicine National Institutes of Health, April 2009. Web.

Pesce, Nicole Lyn. "'10 Day Detox Diet' Author Mark Hyman Tells How to End Sugar Addiction and Clean Up Your Diet." *NYDailyNews.com.* NY Daily News, 11 February 2014. Web.

Rath, Linda. "How Cherries Help Fight Arthritis." *Arthritis.org.* Arthritis Foundation. Web.

Reuters. "Study Finds Cinnamon May Kill E. Coli in Unpasteurized Apple Juice." *LATimes.com.* Los Angeles Times, 6 August 1999. Web.

Ross, Julia. "The Diet Cure." New York: Penguin Publishing Group, 2012. Print.

Sheridan, Mike. "Is Cardio Making You Skinny Fat?" *StrengthSensei.com.* Charles R. Poliquin, 9 March 2015. Web.

Van Cauter, Eva., Knutson, Kristen., et al. "The Impact of Sleep Deprivation on Hormones and Metabolism." *Medscape.org.* Medscape Neurology, 2005. Web.

Volz, Monique. "The Best Gluten Free Chocolate Chip Cookies." *AmbitiousKitchen.com.* Ambitious Kitchen. 25 March 2014. Web.

"What Foods to Avoid?" *MSGTruth.com.* MSGTruth. Web.

Williams, Sara C.P. "Gut Reaction: The Vibrant Ecosystem Inside the Human Gut Does More than Digest Food." *Howard Hughes Medical Institute Bulletin.* (2010): 14-17. Print.

Yang, Qing. "Gain Weight by 'Going Diet?' Artificial Sweeteners and the Neurobiology of Sugar Cravings." *PubMed Central.* US National Library of Medicine National Institutes of Health, June 2010. Web.

ABOUT THE AUTHOR

Linda wants to live in a world where there is an organic coffee shop, a Victoria's Secret, and a gym on every corner. On a more serious note, she wants to live in a world where we, as women, instead of tearing each other down, learn to build each other up, and celebrate one another's differences, thus rising to our fullest potential.

Linda Mitchell is the owner of Chickfit Studio in Mason, Ohio. She enjoys coaching clients, writing, and cooking up "healthy experiments," as her son Jake calls them. She has been married for twenty-one years to Tracy—a very sexy redhead—and has three grown children, Michael, Tiffany, and Jake. At age fifty, Linda became a graduate of the Institute of Integrative Nutrition and an award winning fitness competitor.

Linda is an established writer. As a women's health and fitness expert, she collaborated on the fitness portion of the book *Fat Flush for Life* with mentor and New York Times bestselling author, Ann Louise Gittleman. *Fat Flush for Life* was listed in Time magazine as one of the top ten diet books of 2009. Linda has enjoyed writing her own column "Fit over Forty" for Ms. Fitness magazine for more than a decade. She has also written several magazine articles and cover stories on Suzanne Somers, Dara Torres, Kim Dolan Leto, Nicole Moneer Guerrero, Yoga Fit guru Beth Shaw, basketball superstar Nancy Lieberman, and numerous others.

Linda has made various fitness video and TV appearances on Fox, Fox Sports, WKRC News, WCPO News, WXIX News, and in The Deceptive Diet Plan video.

Linda has coordinated numerous group fitness programs at local health clubs and has conducted personal training for the last thirty years. She is the founder of Chickfit Studio which is specifically devoted to fulfilling the needs of women. After spending time with women from all walks of life, Linda has developed her own philosophies on what works and what doesn't. Linda has many years of experience dealing with women of all ages and fitness levels. One client described her as "the transformation queen" while another declared her to be an "absolute inspiration." She has used the valuable experience that she has learned through competing to help others achieve their ultimate goals and reach their peak performance. Linda believes that there are no limits to the results you can achieve through her hands-on approach and group fitness coaching style.

Linda keeps in touch with the latest industry trends in fitness to keep her training and teaching fresh and current. She is certified in the following: AFAA Personal Training, AFAA Group Fitness Instructor, YogaFit Level 1-5 Instructor, Plyo-Glide, TRX Suspension Training, Kangaroo Cardio using Kangoo Jump Shoes, POSE method running, Roadrunners of America running, AFAA Step Aerobics, Spinning, Zumba, S.T.R.I.D.E., Hip Hop Hustle, Pi-Yo, Turbo Kick, AEA Water Aerobics, SCW Mat Pilates, Kickboxing, and boot camp. Linda is very passionate about Chickfit and has had amazing success through her coaching and classes. Her greatest joy is helping others to achieve their weight loss and fitness goals!

When she's not teaching Chickfit boot camp, you may find Linda at a Fitness America Competition, a Reebok Spartan Race, Surfing, White Water Rafting, listening to Audible while running sprints, or cuddling up on the couch with her husband. This girl really likes to keep it moving.

With over thirty years of experience in the fitness industry under her belt, Linda truly has women's bodies down to a science. Join Linda as she takes you on a fit adventure and transforms your perception of what is possible for you.

Made in the USA
Columbia, SC
17 August 2019